Relief from Snoring and Sleep Apnoea

Tess Graham has successfully delivered
breathing retraining programs to more
than 5000 people. She graduated from the
University of New South Wales with a science
degree, majoring in anatomy and physiology
and achieved a post-graduate qualification in
physiotherapy before taking up professional
practice. For two decades she ran a clinical
practice focused entirely on breathing issues.
Tess now travels in Australia and abroad
speaking on sleep, breathing and health. She
lives in Canberra with her family.

relief from snoring and sleep apnoea

A step-by-step guide to restful sleep
and better health through
changing the way you breathe

TESS GRAHAM

VIKING
an imprint of
PENGUIN BOOKS

PENGUIN BOOKS

UK | USA | Canada | Ireland | Australia
India | New Zealand | South Africa | China

Penguin Books is part of the Penguin Random House group of companies
whose addresses can be found at global.penguinrandomhouse.com.

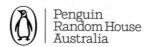

Penguin
Random House
Australia

First published by Penguin Group (UK), 2013
This revised edition published by Penguin Group (Australia), 2014

Text copyright © Tess Graham 2012
Illustrations copyright © Anthony Calvert/The Jacky Winter Group 2012

The moral right of the author has been asserted

Cover design by Alex Ross © Penguin Group (Australia)
Text design by Laura Thomas © Penguin Group (Australia)
Typeset in Minion Pro by Penguin Group (Australia)
Printed and bound in Australia by Griffin Press, an accredited ISO AS/NZS 14001
Environmental Management Systems printer.

National Library of Australia
Cataloguing-in-Publication data:

Graham, Tess.
Relief from snoring and sleep apnoea / Tess Graham.
9780670076499 (pbk.)
Snoring – Prevention.
Sleep apnoea syndromes – Prevention.

616.209

penguin.com.au

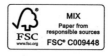

Contents

To my father, Thomas McMahon 1924–2002,
my greatest mentor, and my keenest student

Foreword

BY DR ROSS G. T. WALKER, FRACP, CONSULTANT CARDIOLOGIST

The quality of your day depends on the quality of your sleep the night before. In our society busy schedules may cut in to sleep time, our sleep quality may be affected by our environment, or, as is increasingly more common, we might have a sleep disorder.

As a doctor, I have seen first-hand the devastating effects of snoring and sleep apnoea. The health risks associated with these conditions are well-documented – high blood pressure, increased chance of heart attack or stroke, not to mention the results of a bad night's sleep, such as poor concentration, drowsiness and memory problems. Many sufferers go to great lengths to deal with snoring or sleep apnoea, and yet few understand the role that improved breathing habits can play in managing these disorders.

This isn't just another book about the latest surgical procedures or appliances developed to deal with the problem. Rather, this is an easy-to-read, scientifically based book that justifies a rethink of what is going on for someone with sleep-disordered breathing. It closely examines the differences in the way someone who snores and/or has sleep apnoea breathes, and how someone who sleeps quietly and restfully breathes. And those differences are extraordinary. The potential benefits of breathing retraining – better quality sleep and improved energy levels – are similarly astonishing. By following the program outlined on the following pages, sufferers can experience those differences in their own lives.

In recent times, treatments for snoring and sleep apnoea have focused on technological innovation and intrusive interventions that do not always work, or are not always acceptable or tolerable to the patient. And yet the simplest – and most natural – method of managing these problems has often been overlooked. Going back to the fundamentals of good breathing can make all the difference to what happens when head meets pillow.

I have long been aware of the importance and the health benefits of correct breathing and have witnessed how breathing retraining can restore sound breathing habits and change lives in the process. In fact, if breathing retraining were to be given the place in primary health-care management that it merits, we may well find that the implications for community health and the potential savings to governments would be substantial. Now, in this practical guide, Tess Graham reveals nine habits that can help you to overcome the dysfunctional breathing linked to sleep apnoea and snoring – and you can even get started while you read. Her easy-to-follow five-day program shows you how to breathe the way nature intended – silently, gently and rhythmically.

We can't opt out of breathing. We can do it well, or we can do it poorly. This book is an invaluable resource for those of us determined to maintain or restore good breathing, good health and quality sleep. Tess's program can help you get back to basics with your breathing, and enjoy the improvements to your health and wellbeing.

I, for one, sleep better for having read this book.

Important note

Breathing retraining to improve or normalise dysfunctional breathing is inherently safe. However, if you have any serious illness or significant medical condition requiring ongoing treatment or medication (including psychiatric illness), you should always consult your doctor before undertaking any change to your health management, including undergoing breathing retraining.

Depending on your particular medical circumstances, there may be reasons why you should not seek to make certain changes in your breathing, and there are some people for whom a change in breathing pattern must be approached with some caution. An increased breathing rate, for example, may be part of the body's way of compensating for certain conditions, such as anaemia, diabetes, and emphysema/chronic obstructive pulmonary disorder (COPD). Breathing is also closely linked to body chemistry – blood-sugar levels, for example, can alter with a change in breathing (as they can with a change in diet or amount of physical exercise taken).

It is therefore important if you have any serious illness or significant condition that you make sure all of the changes you are hoping to bring about are suitable for you. Be guided by your doctor – someone who knows your full medical picture. An integrated approach involving your doctor, other healthcare providers, and a knowledgeable and experienced breathing educator may be the best approach when snoring and sleep apnoea are complicated by other significant disorders.

For anyone undergoing breathing retraining, seeing your doctor regularly throughout the process allows him/her to monitor the effects of the changes in your breathing pattern and make decisions regarding medications and prescribed treatments if and when necessary. You should always have your doctor's approval before stopping or modifying any prescribed treatment.

The processes, stories, case studies, client statistics and results presented in this book are from the author's clinical experience. They are not necessarily the processes and results that a reader of this book will experience or achieve. They can only represent the outcome for a particular individual, or the average and typical outcomes of the breathing retraining process in the author's experience.

The author is not engaged to render professional advice or services to the reader. The ideas, procedures and suggestions contained in this book are not intended as a substitute for consulting your medical practitioner. The author is not liable or responsible for any loss or damage arising from any information or suggestions in this book. While the author has used reasonable efforts to ensure the information contained in this book is accurate and up to date the author makes no warranties or representations as to the accuracy of the information and provides no guarantee or promise about the effects and treatment of any health conditions.

Introduction

Read this book and prepare to be shocked. What I am about to show you is a very different way of looking at snoring, sleep apnoea and poor sleep.

The first thing you should know is that if you snore or have sleep apnoea, you are not breathing correctly. No exceptions! People who breathe correctly do not snore or have sleep apnoea. The good news is you can change your breathing. But first you have to know what needs changing.

Have you ever heard that it is best to breathe deeply, fully and even forcefully? In with the good air, out with the bad, right? If you think this is good for you, you are not alone – but you need to think again. Ironically, this is how most snorers breathe, and often it is how someone with sleep apnoea breathes just before their throat collapses!

You may be one of the many who believe that having surgery or wearing a dental appliance or a mask and air pump to bed each night are the only ways to get relief from snoring and sleep apnoea. You also may have been advised to get fit and lose weight. While all these approaches can certainly help, very few people are aware of what I believe may be the most effective approach of all – breathing retraining.

By learning to breathe more gently, smoothly and efficiently you can significantly improve your sleep and your health, boost your energy levels, and subsequently improve your quality of life.

In this book you'll discover what correct breathing is and how to achieve it. You will be delighted by just how simple making these changes can be and perhaps even a little surprised to learn that good breathing is the opposite of what you think. You will read about lives having been transformed, just by learning to breathe properly.

Take Bill, for example.

At age 48, Bill sometimes wondered if he was going to die early, or at least have to give up work. His twenty-year-plus snoring problem had deteriorated into sleep apnoea – where his horrendous snoring was now interrupted by worrying silences, then gasping and choking episodes as he resumed breathing. Sometimes Bill woke himself up with particularly loud snoring or the jerking of his body as he fought for his breathing to resume. His days were punctuated by nausea, diarrhoea, and unbelievable fatigue. Fainting was the final straw, and Bill went to see his doctor.

An overnight sleep study showed that Bill had moderately severe sleep apnoea. He was advised to have laser surgery to remove a portion of his soft palate. The other option was to use a CPAP machine – an air pump attached to a face mask. However, Bill was not guaranteed that surgery was a permanent solution nor that it would solve his particular problem, and he learnt that some spouses of CPAP wearers found the appliance very intrusive.

It was a stroke of good luck for Bill that while faced with this difficult choice, he heard about a breathing retraining course. The concept made sense to him – after all, for over two decades there obviously had been something wrong with the way he was breathing! From the second day of the breathing course he noticed an improvement in his sleep. By the end of that week his concentration and stamina were better, and according to his wife, there was no more snoring. Some months later he had a repeat sleep study done – there was no evidence of sleep apnoea. By taking responsibility for the way he breathed, Bill had in effect 'fixed' himself.

We take for granted our ability to breathe. But we can breathe well, or we can breathe poorly. Snoring, sleep apnoea, asthma, chronic mouth-breathing, stuffy noses and a lot of other common conditions involve *disordered* breathing.

Relief from Snoring and Sleep Apnoea is about recognising this. It shows you how to regain control over a basic life force: your breath. It provides you with an easy, simple and natural way to achieve your dream of having quiet, restful, refreshing sleep night after night. How? Simply by learning to breathe correctly.

There are two parts to this book. Part one is about awareness. It guides you through the process of assessing your baseline breathing pattern, and if you are a snorer or have sleep apnoea, you will be left in little doubt that you are breathing incorrectly. You will also learn what you need to change in order to breathe and sleep better. I will help you understand the connection between your pattern of breathing and snoring, apnoea, stuffy nose, an inflamed throat, jerking limbs, a thumping headache on waking, anxiety, debilitating day-long fatigue, poor concentration and myriad other symptoms associated with snoring and sleep apnoea.

Part two is the program itself. It is a practical guide to changing your breathing; learning to breathe again the way you did when you did not snore. Here I'll tell you about the habits you need to cultivate to improve your breathing – the nine healthy breathing habits that I have seen quickly restore quality sleep, energy and a great sense of wellbeing to my clients.

We have much to thank modern medicine for, but I believe there is a price to pay when we rely on it too heavily and fail to look to ourselves for solutions to our health problems. In the past, we have been inclined to overemphasise the idea of there being a magic bullet, or to wait for the next medical miracle to come along. Today, however, it is widely accepted that much chronic illness is preventable through better lifestyle choices, and modern medicine in conjunction with the popular media, has made us much more aware of the importance to health of diet and exercise.

To this we must add breathing well.

This book is based on solid scientific principles and research evidence, but I have simplified the explanations of physiology and biochemistry for a lay audience – at the end of the book are reference and research materials for those who want to delve more deeply into the scientific detail. The examples, stories, case studies and 'before and after' figures come from my many years of clinical practice. The names I have used are fictitious; the experiences are real. The stories may be individual experiences, or composites of typical real-life experiences that I have witnessed over and over again, scores if not hundreds of times. I hope they will enlighten, inspire and reassure you that you are not alone; that you are not 'a hopeless case'. They demonstrate that improving the way you breathe is eminently doable and infinitely rewarding.

Although the principles of breathing retraining apply to both adults and children, the program described in this book is more suitable for adults and children fourteen years and over. However, younger children can be helped by what their parents learn and can be encouraged to try the basic practices that require less focus. And while the book is specifically written for people with sleep-breathing issues, the information contained here may be of help to anyone suffering from conditions that are breathing-related. I have worked with Olympic athletes, social exercisers, the sedentary, the physically disabled; singers and actors; men, women and children of all ages. It was breathing retraining that twenty years ago freed my children from the grip of asthma and became the turning point in my career.

The book takes into account our time-poor, fast-paced world. You will be shown how to blend breathing retraining into your daily activities, including physical exercise. The aim is to make good breathing your new way of being rather than something to be practised only when you get around to it. Before the end of Part two, you will be on your way to breathing and sleeping better. Some change is generally apparent within 24 hours, with benefits increasing over time as your breathing pattern improves and becomes second nature.

This book presents you with an opportunity to empower yourself and improve your health and the quality of your life. Like so many before you, you may even get your old life back – the one you thought was gone forever.

PART ONE
UNDERSTANDING SNORING AND SLEEP APNOEA: THE WAY YOU BREATHE, THE SLEEP YOU GET

'Life is a perpetual instruction in cause and effect.'

RALPH WALDO EMERSON

CHAPTER 1

Snoring and sleep apnoea – what are they?

There are many different types of sleep disorders and they may be linked to various medical conditions. The focus of this book is those related to a disturbed or disordered breathing pattern during sleep – they are called *sleep-breathing disorders*; they involve *sleep-disordered breathing*. Snoring and sleep apnoea are two forms of sleep-disordered breathing. They are unfortunately well known to many households throughout the developed world. Not only does sleep-disordered breathing deprive you of quality sleep, but it predisposes you to a number of serious health conditions. It may also have profound social repercussions – relationships and job performance can suffer.

WHAT IS SNORING?

Snoring is noisy and often uneven breathing that occurs during sleep. The typical snoring noise is made while breathing in, and it comes from vibration of 'soft' tissues in the nose and throat. If you snore and have a partner then you will surely know about it! The noise can vary from a soft purr to a sound similar to a semitrailer using its airbrakes. The average noise level of snorers is 60 decibels. (Normal speech range is 40 to 60 decibels.) A really loud snorer can reach 90 decibels, a level that could be hazardous to your hearing.

Around 40 per cent of the adult population snores at least occasionally, with the figure rising to an estimated 60 per cent in the over 40s. While the incidence is greater in men, more than 30 per cent of middle-aged women habitually snore. Worsening snoring is a risk factor for developing obstructive sleep apnoea – around 50 per cent of middle-aged habitual snorers could have obstructive sleep apnoea. (When someone just snores and does not have sleep apnoea it is called *simple snoring*.) Snoring is also common in children.

WHAT IS SLEEP APNOEA?

Sleep apnoea is where breathing stops during sleep for more than ten seconds at a time, five or more times per hour, accompanied by a drop in the level of oxygen in the blood and disruption to sleep. (The word *apnoea* or *apnea* comes from the Greek: 'a' meaning 'lack of' and 'pnoea' meaning 'to breathe'.) Sleep can be disrupted hundreds of times in just one night, and sufferers may be prevented from entering or spending adequate time in the deep, restorative sleep stage. Blood pressure can increase and there are changes in heart rate and rhythm associated with apnoea episodes.

Apnoea is followed by waking, semi-wakening or an *arousal*. An arousal is an abrupt change from deep sleep to lighter sleep. Arousals are typically so brief that they are not remembered the next morning. The longer apnoeas, though, may fully wake the person with a sharp jolt, a frightening feeling of choking, or even of drowning. Not surprisingly, the sufferer does not feel well rested the next day.

There are three forms of sleep apnoea.

Obstructive sleep apnoea (OSA)

Obstructive sleep apnoea, the most common type, is where the person stops breathing because of an obstruction in their upper airway, typically in the pharynx – the wall of the throat behind the nose and tongue. There are degrees of severity. Typically the apnoea interrupts a period of loud snoring with 10–90 seconds of silence. The breathing muscles continue to work hard, trying to inhale through the blocked airway.

This struggle to breathe eventually causes the person to arouse momentarily, the throat opens, and they breathe again and fall back asleep. There is typically a snort or gasp and their whole body shudders as they arouse. (With severe obstructive sleep apnoea there are more than 30 'events' like this per hour.)

Snoring almost always occurs with obstructive apnoea, although not everybody who snores will have apnoea.

Central sleep apnoea (CSA)

In central sleep apnoea, breathing stops during sleep when the *central nervous system* (the brain) temporarily stops transmitting signals to the breathing muscles. All breathing movements stop temporarily, typically for 30–60 seconds. Central sleep apnoea can be caused by a number of conditions that influence the breathing-control centre – the *respiratory centre* – in the brain. Central apnoea is less frequently diagnosed than the obstructive form and may often go unrecognised. Central apnoea can occur without snoring.

Mixed or complex sleep apnoea

Mixed sleep apnoea is a combination of obstructive and central sleep apnoea. This may also be termed *complex sleep apnoea*.

Other associated conditions

Associated with sleep apnoea are two other conditions. *Hypopnoea* is where breathing is reduced significantly but does not stop completely. ('Hypo' is from the Greek word for 'under'.) *Upper airway resistance syndrome* (UARS) is where there is narrowing of the upper airway and increased resistance to airflow, but without any significant periods of breathing stoppage. There can be snoring, gasping and repetitive arousals. The episodes of narrowing and arousal can occur hundreds of times per night.

SLEEP APNOEA ON THE RISE

The incidence of sleep apnoea is increasing. Estimates of the number of people suffering from sleep apnoea vary: it is believed that most people with obstructive sleep apnoea are not diagnosed, and central sleep apnoea may occur without symptoms.

As with snoring, the incidence of obstructive apnoea is higher in males and more common in the overweight and middle-aged. The prevalence of symptomatic obstructive sleep apnoea has been variously estimated between 1 and 6 per cent in the adult population.[1.1] A 2000 report from Australia's National Health and Medical Research Council (NHMRC) quotes one source as identifying clinically significant obstructive sleep apnoea in 24 per cent of men and 6 per cent of women over 55.[1.2]

The American National Sleep Foundation estimates that more than 18 million American adults have sleep apnoea and that a minimum prevalence of 2 to 3 per cent exists in children.[1.3]

The implications of these conditions can reverberate (as does heavy snoring) far and wide beyond the bedroom.

CHAPTER 2

The dangers of snoring and sleep apnoea

Snoring is a lot more than just a noise hazard. You can wake with a dry mouth, bad breath and a headache similar to a hangover, but without the party the night before. You can wake feeling more tired than when you went to bed. If snoring makes sleep restless and fragmented through frequent waking and jostling around, it impairs your functioning the next day. This can show in low energy, feeling sleepy, slowed reflexes and impaired thinking and reasoning ability. Similar symptoms are seen with upper airway resistance syndrome.

While snoring has long been the butt of many jokes, habitual snoring needs to be taken seriously – even if it is classified in the 'non-divorce-able' category – as over time it may progress to heavier snoring. There is a high incidence of chronic snoring among men who suffer strokes. Heavy snoring is also associated with an increased incidence of high blood pressure and heart attack.

Women who snore during pregnancy have a higher incidence of pre-eclampsia – pregnancy-related high blood pressure – and babies with low birth weight and low Apgar scores. (The Apgar score is used to assess a baby's health immediately after birth.) A significant number of heavy snorers report reduced sexual drive (their fatigued bed partners are also likely to experience this). It is also quite common for male snorers to experience erectile dysfunction.

Heavy snoring can be an early manifestation of the much more serious obstructive sleep apnoea. Untreated sleep apnoea puts you at greater risk for some serious health disorders, including the following:

- high blood pressure
- irregular heart rhythms and heart attacks
- sexual dysfunction
- reflux/heartburn
- depression
- obesity
- stroke
- angina
- sleep deprivation
- diabetes
- cancer.

There is also increasing recognition of the contribution of driver fatigue to road accidents (it is suspected to be a major factor in up to 40 per cent of road accidents).[2.1] People with obstructive sleep apnoea are said to be two to seven times more likely than people without sleep apnoea to have a road accident.[2.2] They also have an increased incidence of workplace accidents. Sleep deprivation from any cause is a concern – simple snoring as well as sleep apnoea can contribute to daytime sleepiness.

HEALTH HAZARDS FOR YOUR OTHER HALF

Partners of snorers and sleep apnoea sufferers often have poor sleep, fatigue, irritability and concentration problems. A Mayo Clinic study indicated they can lose around an hour of sleep per night.[2.3] Their sleep can be quite fragmented – they can wake at least briefly around twenty times an hour.[2.4] They may shove, pull, punch and kick their partner in the hope that repositioning them will solve the problem.

> For three consecutive years, Christine had fronted up for her annual medical examination with her only complaint being that she was feeling terribly tired. She needed a nap every day, and every evening she was so tired that she wanted to cry. Her doctor had run all the blood tests and could find nothing wrong with her. Then Christine said, 'Maybe my problem is my snoring husband?' Turns out, she was right.

AND THAT'S NOT ALL...

Snoring can be a major embarrassment to the snorer, and a major annoyance for others who share the room or even the house. Relationships can suffer. Many couples blame their rows on snoring and some have considered splitting up as a way of escaping persistent snoring. In fact, snoring is said to be the third biggest cause of marriage breakdowns.

Many couples in which one partner snores sleep in separate bedrooms. Sleep deprivation is probably also behind an emerging trend in new home construction. A BBC news item in 2007 reported that more and more new homes in America are being built with two master bedrooms.[2.4]

Snoring can also have repercussions at work. Job performance can suffer due to low energy, poor concentration and impaired reflexes and reasoning ability. Persistent daytime sleepiness, including nodding off at inappropriate times, could threaten job security.

But all is not lost. If you have ever slept soundly, breathing quietly and rhythmically, then you can most likely get back to that breathing pattern again.

CHAPTER 3

How do you know if you have sleep-disordered breathing?

To understand these modern 'epidemics', and in particular your own breathing issues, we need to learn a little about sleep itself, then look at what can go wrong during it. Sleep is a natural state of rest for the mind and body, and vitally important for health and wellbeing. It is as crucial as air, food and water. It recharges you, supports your immune system and helps supply you with the mental, emotional and physical energy to get through the day.

Sleep occurs in cyclical stages characterised by different patterns of electrical activity in the brain, including periods of lighter and deeper sleep and periods of dreaming.

These different stages are important components of restful and restorative sleep. Many of the body's functions and hormones have a pattern of rise and fall that depends upon the cyclical patterns of day and night, of wakefulness and sleep. Sleep well and you wake refreshed, with energy to burn.

If your sleep is impaired in any way, you can really suffer for it, mentally and physically. Poor sleep impacts your levels of thyroid and stress hormones, your immune system, metabolism, mood, brain function and energy. It's even linked to laying down abdominal fat and an increased risk of diabetes.

If you wake up tired, most of your sleep probably occurred in the lighter sleep stages, with you missing out on the deeper, recuperative sleep stages. This is common with sleep apnoea.

Even one night of disrupted sleep can lead to difficulty getting up in the morning, irritability, poor concentration and slow decision-making. Energy can be low, reflexes slow, and you can be clumsy and sleepy. You may look to prop yourself up with potentially harmful amounts of stimulants like caffeine and energy drinks. You may put yourself, your family and others at risk too – staying awake for just one night can impair your ability to drive, in a similar way to as if you were intoxicated.

BREATHING DURING SLEEP
What is normal?
Breathing moves air in and out of the body. The main function of the breathing process is to bring about the exchange of two gases – oxygen and carbon dioxide – and to maintain them at the optimal levels.

Normal breathing during sleep is silent, and in and out through the nose – similar to normal daytime breathing. The pattern changes a little between the different sleep stages but is generally smooth and gentle. During sleep however, the body is deeply at rest and the volume of air being breathed is (for the most part) naturally lower than it is in the day.[3.1, 3.2] Warmth can be felt at the nose, but not 'wind'. In other words, normal breathing during sleep should be just as quiet and gentle, if not more so, than when you are awake.

A normal breather falls asleep within a few minutes, sleeps the whole night without awakening, does not move about much, and wakes fully refreshed after seven hours or so.

Sleep-disordered breathing
The term *sleep-disordered breathing* describes any abnormal pattern of breathing occurring during sleep. Examples include snoring, snorting, erratic breathing, stop-start breathing, apnoea and hypopnoea. The breathing pattern is uneven, and the volume of air moving in and out can vary from a gale during heavy snoring to nothing during apnoea – and everything in between.

FIGURE 3.1: NORMAL BREATHING DURING SLEEP

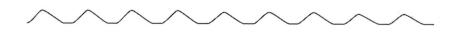

FIGURE 3.2: TYPICAL PATTERN SEEN WITH OBSTRUCTIVE SLEEP APNOEA

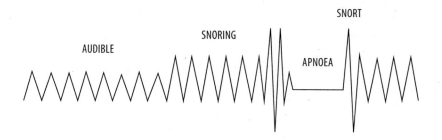

A person with snoring and sleep apnoea may breathe two to three times more air than the norm – when they *are* breathing! As well as being noisy, this dries out the mouth and throat. They may sleep eight to ten, even twelve, hours, tossing and turning often, with leg movements and frequently disrupted sleep throughout the night. Despite the longer sleep, they wake feeling totally unrefreshed; in fact, more tired than before bed. If that's how you feel after sleep, how will you feel at the end of a day's work?

HOW ARE SLEEP-BREATHING DISORDERS DIAGNOSED?

Diagnosis takes into consideration the symptoms experienced by the sufferer, reports from family members and the findings of physical examinations and various testing procedures. People with sleep-disordered breathing often go to see their doctor because they are tired all the time or because a sleep partner or roommate complains about their snoring and/or has observed breaks in their breathing and gasping episodes.

Although a person with sleep apnoea usually sleeps through apnoea episodes, they may become aware of the problem because they wake themselves with a particularly loud snore or snort, or a choking feeling, or through the jerking of their body as they struggle to resume breathing. Initially, however, they can be unaware of the real nature and extent of their breathing difficulties during sleep.

David, 54, was a shocking snorer, according to his family. Relatives staying overnight knew to bring earplugs. It was his wife who made him see his doctor. She was frightened because David repeatedly stopped breathing each night. She would try to hold her breath as long as he did and couldn't. David had no idea how serious it was for him, but he did find his restless legs very disturbing. He would be moving them about, trying to relieve the pain even though he was exhausted and needed to sleep. At times, David would wake himself up gasping for air or with his own loud snorting, but would immediately go back to sleep. He did not realise he had sleep apnoea.

Here is a list of signs and symptoms that may indicate someone has sleep apnoea:

- loud snoring
- gagging, gasping or choking episodes during sleep
- sudden awakenings with a snort
- restless sleep, sleep interruptions
- twitching of the legs or arms during sleep
- an irresistible urge to move the legs just before or during sleep ('restless legs')
- waking up feeling tired and groggy
- morning headache
- breathlessness (day or night)
- feeling depressed, anxious, moody, or irritable
- symptoms of sleep deprivation, such as:
  - ▸ daytime sleepiness
  - ▸ low energy, always feeling tired
  - ▸ falling asleep at inappropriate times

▸ slower reaction time – driving car or using work machinery
▸ poor concentration and short-term memory
▸ impaired thinking, judgement and reasoning ability
▸ decreased productivity.

Typically someone with sleep apnoea wakes in the morning feeling incredibly tired, often with a feeling of a hangover, a headache, a mouth like the bottom of a birdcage, and a fatigued and aching body. Generally the symptoms develop over years and may be seen to progress with increasing weight and stress levels. Symptoms may appear with the onset of menopause in women. A diagnosis of sleep apnoea should be suspected in people who are obese, have high blood pressure, snore and have daytime sleepiness.

Eventually sleepiness interferes with work and reduces quality of life – the symptoms of sleep deprivation can become very much a part of your life. (Significant fatigue can be experienced by heavy snorers even if they do not have apnoea.) Other symptoms associated with sleep apnoea include waking with your heart racing or pounding, sweating, heartburn/reflux, reduced sex drive, impotence, thirst, repeated need to urinate at night, bedwetting in children, insomnia and waking with a dry, sore throat (please see Important note, page 32). Restless legs syndrome has been linked to several serious illnesses including hypothyroidism, diabetes and kidney disease. See your doctor to be checked for these conditions if you suffer from restless legs. Restlessness and twitching in muscles is also, however, a well-known symptom of disordered breathing and generally responds well to breathing training.

There are a variety of tools that your doctor may use for diagnosis including questionnaires to assess daytime sleepiness, physical examination, X-ray and MRI scans of the nose, mouth and throat, and sleep studies.

Physical examination by your family doctor or ear, nose and throat (ENT) specialist may look for signs of airway swelling and narrowing, such as nasal polyps – small sac-like growths of inflamed nasal tissue – or an enlarged uvula, tonsils or adenoids. Tonsils and adenoids are glands –

tonsils are in the throat, and the adenoids sit at the back of the nose. The uvula is the punching bag–shaped piece of tissue hanging from the back of your soft palate. The palate, in the roof of the mouth, consists of the hard palate at the front of the mouth, which contains bone, and the soft palate at the back, which does not contain bone. If your doctor suspects sleep apnoea, you will likely be referred for an overnight sleep study.

Polysomnography (or sleep study) is sleep medicine's 'gold standard' for diagnosis of sleep disorders. Leads and sensors are applied to various parts of the body to monitor its activities during sleep, including brain and heart rhythms, chest and abdominal movements, leg movement, sleep position, oxygen levels, snoring levels, arousals, airflow and periods of apnoea. The data is analysed by a computer and a report prepared. Five or more apnoea or hypopnoea episodes per hour is regarded as abnormal; more than fifteen episodes per hour is rated as moderately severe sleep apnoea; more than 30 per hour is classified as severe.

The demand for sleep studies has risen dramatically in the last decade. The long waiting lists and associated costs for studies done in hospitals, specialised sleep clinics and laboratories have led to the development of home-diagnosis equipment.

This would seem to be a positive development as your sleeping pattern in the privacy and comfort of your own bed is likely to better represent your usual sleep than that in the artificial environment of a sleep lab. Some people find their sleep in the lab is disturbed by the wires attached to their body, the noise of air-conditioners, the room tempera-ture and the movements of technicians. (I've known of people who got up and left in the middle of the night!)

Though the home sleep studies offer considerable benefits in terms of cost, convenience and availability, the quality of diagnostic information may not be as high as in a laboratory study.

AN ADDITIONAL PERSPECTIVE

What I propose in this book is that an abnormal pattern of breathing is likely to be a primary factor in your snoring and sleep apnoea – although anatomical and other factors may well compound the problem for many.

I believe, therefore, routine assessment of a person's baseline breathing pattern to be a very important addition to the diagnostic procedures currently in use.

When someone who snores and/or has sleep apnoea comes to see a breathing educator, an essential first step is observation and assessment of their breathing pattern. The breathing educator looks for signs of disturbance in the normal rhythm, rate and volume of breathing, the way the breathing muscles are used and whether mouth- or nose-breathing is favoured. These factors are very important, because the way you breathe during sleep is a reflection of your breathing pattern/habits during the day. Critically, there is an association between the amount of air you breathe per second and per minute and the potential to snore and trigger apnoea. There is also an association between mouth-breathing and the incidence of apnoea.

Identifying just how someone's breathing pattern differs from normal, healthy breathing lights the way back to better breathing habits and quiet, restful sleep. Let's check yours now.

CHAPTER 4

Know your breathing 24/7

How should you breathe? How does a silent, restful sleeper breathe? How does a snorer or person with sleep apnoea breathe? Do they only breathe badly when asleep? Most importantly, how do you breathe? There are some simple observations you can make at home to determine if your breathing pattern is normal or not.

What you may not realise is that your breathing does not just go berserk during sleep before returning to a perfectly normal pattern when you wake up. While your breathing can get considerably worse when you are asleep, it in fact reflects how you breathe during the day. It is also a reflection of the 'set point' of the respiratory centre in your brain – the target level for carbon dioxide in the blood that it tries to maintain. If you breathe incorrectly over a certain period of time, you can alter this setting.

The way you are breathing right now could be making you sick, tired and dopey and be preparing you (and your partner) for a rough and noisy night. Breath by breath, likely 20 000 times a day, you could be disturbing your blood gases and chemistry and interfering with the function of every system in your body.

First, we will look at how you are breathing now, then how you breathe at night, then at which symptoms of disordered or dysfunctional breathing you may be experiencing. Please note that this is a check that you can do yourself on certain aspects of your *breathing pattern* and on your *breathing habits*. It is quite different from the breathing tests (spirometry) commonly used in doctors' surgeries and hospitals to diagnose and assess asthma and COPD. It also differs from the technical overnight sleep studies used to diagnose and evaluate the severity of sleep-breathing disorders.

Do not, however, be fooled by the simplicity of this self-assessment process. It helps you to check things about your breathing pattern that may not have been checked before. It is important to identify faulty breathing habits as they can set off a cascade of symptoms and may well underlie nasal and sleep-breathing problems. People rarely focus on their breathing as it is innate and automatic and so they are often unaware of their poor breathing habits. You may indeed be surprised at what you are about to discover.

BREATHING PATTERN SELF-ASSESSMENT – DAYTIME

First you will assess your usual daytime breathing pattern. You will need a timer or watch with a second hand, and two different coloured pens. Record your observations in Table 4.1 (page 19). (An alternative is to download the free workbook at www.BreatheAbility.com, which has all the tables and checklists you need to complete.)

Instructions for completing Table 4.1
1.   Write today's date at the top of the Assessment 1 column.
2.   Spend a few moments observing your breathing according to the guidelines below. Try not to alter it in any way, just observe. *Pay no attention to any preconceived ideas of how you should be breathing.*
3.   For each of the parameters/elements of breathing, record your observations in column 1 – using the number, the percentage or the particular word or words that apply to you.

The parameters
'FEEL' OF YOUR BREATHING
Does your breathing feel easy (satisfying), or heavy (laboured), restricted, or do you feel breathless?

TABLE 4.1: BREATHING PATTERN SELF-ASSESSMENT – DAYTIME

BREATHING PARAMETER	ASSESSMENT 1 Date:	ASSESSMENT 2 Date:	ASSESSMENT 3 Date:
FEEL of BREATHING Easy or heavy /restricted / breathless			
RHYTHM Regular or irregular (erratic / sighing / yawning / throat clearing/ breath holding / coughing)			
SOUND of BREATHING Rest: silent or audible Daily activity: silent or audible Physical exercise: fairly quiet or noisy			
RESPIRATION RATE (Breaths per minute)			
ROUTE: NOSE or MOUTH Rest: nose [%]; mouth [%] Daily activity: nose [%]; mouth [%] Physical exercise: nose [%]; mouth [%]			
POSTURE Upright or slumped			
LOCATION OF BREATHING MOVEMENT Diaphragm / upper chest / shoulders / abdomen *Underline dominant area*			
AIRFLOW Scale 1–4			
HEART RATE (beats/min)			

RHYTHM

Is your breathing regular (flows with a smooth, even pattern), or irregular (erratic timing, variable breath sizes – sighs, yawns, extra-deep breaths, throat clearing, coughs)? Do you find yourself holding your breath at times? Have others ever commented that you sigh a lot?

SOUND OF YOUR BREATHING

There are three situations to consider here.

Rest: Can you hear yourself breathing now – is your breathing silent or audible? Audible means any sound you make as you breathe in and out, as well as any extra-noisy breaths such as throat clearing, sniffing or gasping. Have others commented that they can hear your breathing when sitting beside you watching television or at the cinema? Has anyone ever commented about how heavy your breathing sounds over the phone?

Daily activity: When you are moving about, going upstairs, or lifting something, is your breathing silent or audible? If you're not sure, go and try something now.

Physical exercise: When you are at the gym, walking fast, or playing team sport, is your breathing fairly quiet or is it noisy? Have you ever noticed that your breathing is noisier than that of others?

RESPIRATION RATE

One breath cycle consists of an in-breath (inhalation) and an out-breath (exhalation). Using a watch, count the number of complete breath cycles that you take in one minute (see Figure 4.1, page 21). This will be your *respiration rate*.

Try not to influence its rate while you check this – often your breathing will slow when you try to count the rate yourself. Your 'real' respiration rate could be an extra one to four breaths a minute.

Asking someone else to check it later when you are not aware (e.g., while you are reading or watching TV) may give a more accurate measurement.

FIGURE 4.1: BREATHS PER MINUTE – RESPIRATION RATE

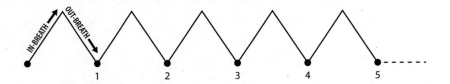

ROUTE: NOSE- OR MOUTH-BREATHING

You will need to estimate the percentage of time you breathe through your nose and the percentage of time you breathe through your mouth in the following three situations.

Rest: Are you breathing through your nose or mouth right now? When sitting, standing or when deep in concentration, what percentage of time do you nose-breathe/mouth-breathe?

Daily activity: When walking about (e.g., shopping), or doing light activities, what percentage of time do you nose-breathe/mouth-breathe?

Physical exercise: During mild–moderate exercise, such as brisk walking, working out at the gym, or playing tennis, what percentage of time do you nose-breathe/mouth-breathe?

These details are often unknown but are very important. I suggest you make a guess now, and then watch yourself closely over the next couple of days and adjust the estimates as necessary.

Most people grossly underestimate the amount of time that they mouth-breathe. Someone else might be able to help you with these observations.

POSTURE

Don't move! Or if you just did after seeing the word 'posture', please move back to your usual sitting posture. Now, without moving your torso, place the thumb of one hand on the lower end of your breastbone and the little finger of the same hand on your navel.

With an upright posture, there is usually a full stretched hand span between these two points. With a slumped posture these two points are brought closer together, with a folding or wrinkling effect of the abdomen. Is your posture upright or slumped (see Figure 4.2)?

FIGURE 4.2: IS YOUR POSTURE SLUMPED OR UPRIGHT?

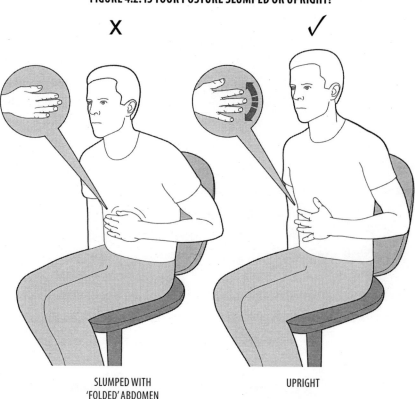

SLUMPED WITH   UPRIGHT
'FOLDED' ABDOMEN

LOCATION OF BREATHING MOVEMENT

To assess how you usually breathe, it is very important that you sit how you usually sit – slumped or otherwise – while making the following observations. Which part(s) of your torso move when you breathe? Notice where you feel the movement or expansion as you breathe in (see Figure 4.3). Do you feel your shoulders or collarbones rise? Do you feel movement of your upper chest and breastbone area, your diaphragm-solar plexus area (above the navel), or your lower abdomen below the navel? You may feel movement in one, several or all of these areas.

Write down in Table 4.1 all the parts that move. Closing your eyes for a minute may help you to better detect where the movements are.

Now place your left hand horizontally across your breastbone and your right hand horizontally across your solar plexus with the little finger above the level of your navel. When you breathe in, does your left hand (chest) or right hand (diaphragm) move first? Which moves the most? In the table, underline either chest or diaphragm to indicate which you feel is the dominant movement.

Once again, asking someone else to observe your breathing when you are not paying attention to it may be helpful in determining your usual manner of breathing.

FIGURE 4.3: UPPER-CHEST BREATHER OR DIAPHRAGM-BREATHER?

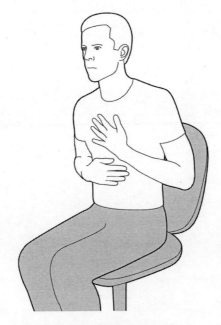

WHICH HAND MOVES FIRST?

AIRFLOW

Place the palm of your hand 1–2 cm in front of and facing your mouth, so that you are just touching the tip of your nose. Rate the degree of airflow you feel on your hand during the out-breath using the scale below. If you sometimes mouth-breathe and sometimes nose-breathe, then assess the flow for each.

Airflow scale: 1 = sensation of warmth, not flow; 2 = gentle flow of air; 3 = definite stream of air; 4 = strong airstream or 'wind'.

HEART RATE OR PULSE AT REST

Strange as it may seem, your breathing affects your heart rate. Just how and why will become clearer later. Take your pulse now and record the number of beats per minute in Table 4.1.

Taking your pulse: You count the pulse on the thumb side of the underside of your wrist about 1–2 cm below the crease line at the base of your hand and 1 cm in from the edge of your wrist. Use two fingers from your other hand and place them gently in the position where you feel the slight throb of the heartbeat. Count the number of beats, or pulses, in one minute.

You have now rated your baseline breathing pattern. It is really interesting to compare the results after you have worked through some strategies to improve your breathing. Bookmark page 19 so you can find it easily.

BREATHING PATTERN ASSESSMENT – ASLEEP

Next, you will rate your usual night-time breathing pattern. For most of the parameters described below you will need to get feedback from someone, as you may be unaware of what is going on when you are asleep. You could ask a bed partner or someone you have shared a campsite or a room with when travelling – that's if you are still on speaking terms!

Instructions for completing Table 4.2

1. Write today's date at the top of the Assessment 1 column of Table 4.2 (page 26).
2. Those who are not using an appliance during sleep complete only the 'No Appliance' column for a typical night.
3. Those who do use an appliance during sleep (e.g., oral/dental splint,

continuous positive airway pressure (CPAP) machine with mask) complete both the With Appliance and the No Appliance columns for each parameter for a typical night. In the No Appliance column you are rating your breathing for what a typical night was like before you got your appliance or when you happen not to use your appliance – for example, while on a camping trip or when you fall asleep on the couch, or if you do not put it back on after a disturbance at night. A 'significant other' can help with this.

4. For some parameters, you may need to record several words in the boxes.

The parameters

RHYTHM

Is your breathing regular (smooth) or irregular (erratic/jerky, varying breath sizes and rates, pauses in breathing, snorts, gasps)? (Please see Important note, page 32.)

SOUND OF YOUR BREATHING

Is your breathing silent, audible or loud? Audible means anything from just a rhythmical sound to snoring, snorting or gasping noises. Loud means your breathing can be heard outside the bedroom.

ROUTE: NOSE- OR MOUTH-BREATHING

Do you breathe predominantly through your mouth or nose while you are asleep? Waking with a dry mouth can indicate mouth-breathing. So can the habit of taking water to bed to sip throughout the night. Your partner may be able to help you estimate the percentage of nose-breathing versus mouth-breathing.

AIRFLOW

If you have a partner, ask them to rate the airflow at your nose or mouth by placing their hand a few centimetres away from your face when you are asleep. Rate the flow of air on the out-breath on a scale of 1–4. (You cannot do this rating if using a CPAP machine.)

Ask your partner if they have felt a stream of air or a breeze blowing on them in bed. If so, they don't need to do the airflow check – it's obviously a 4.

Airflow scale: 1 = sensation of warmth, not flow; 2 = gentle flow of air; 3 = definite stream of air; 4 = strong airstream or 'wind'.

HEART RATE ON WAKING

Your heart rate should generally be at its lowest on waking. It is affected, however, by your overnight breathing. Check it tomorrow as soon as you wake, preferably before you get out of bed.

Bookmark this page so you can come back to it later.

TABLE 4.2: BREATHING PATTERN ASSESSMENT – ASLEEP

BREATHING PARAMETER	ASSESSMENT 1 Date:		ASSESSMENT 2 Date:	ASSESSMENT 3 Date:
	NO APPLIANCE	WITH APPLIANCE Type:		
RHYTHM Regular or irregular (erratic / variable / pauses / gasping / snorting)				
SOUND of BREATHING Silent or audible / loud				
ROUTE: NOSE or MOUTH Nose [%]; Mouth [%]				
AIRFLOW Scale 1–4				
HEART RATE on waking (beats/min)				

Additional information: (tick for yes)

☐ Do you snore in any position?
☐ Do you snore only when lying on your back?
☐ Is your snoring worse when you are on your back?
☐ Is your sleep more disrupted when sleeping on your back?

The next step is to identify symptoms you are experiencing that may be connected to the way you breathe.

SIGNS AND SYMPTOMS OF DYSFUNCTIONAL BREATHING

Snoring, apnoea, fatigue and daytime sleepiness are very rarely the only signs and symptoms displayed by people with sleep-disordered breathing. You may be surprised to learn how many manifestations of dysfunctional breathing you actually have – some of which may appear at first to be totally unrelated to breathing.

Filling out Table 4.3 (pages 30–31) can help you realise the extent to which dysfunctional breathing is affecting your life and the importance of addressing your breathing problems. Some people will have the majority of the items on the list in Table 4.3, others only a few. Many of my clients have more than twenty. It is helpful if you can ask a companion to assist you in identifying and rating the intensity of any snoring, breathing irregularities in sleep, and how restless and interrupted your sleep is.

SCORING SYSTEM:

Empty box	You don't have this symptom, or haven't experienced it during the past week.
✓	An occasional symptom, does not happen every day nor every time you are in a 'trigger' situation. For example, you occasionally fall asleep watching television but do not do it every evening.
✓ ✓	A frequent symptom, present part of most days or nights. For example, you yawn a lot most afternoons; you wake with achy legs four to six times a week.
✓ ✓ ✓	Very frequent symptom, present most of each day or night or whenever in a trigger situation. For example, your nose is at least partly congested most of the day, and always gets worse when you lie down at night.
✓ ✓ ✓ ✓	Very frequent and/or strong symptom. For example, you snore very heavily most of the night.

Instructions for completing Table 4.3

- Write today's date at the top of the Assessment 1 column of Table 4.3.
- Put an X in the 'My Symptoms' column next to those symptoms you *currently* experience at least once a week.
- Now rate the intensity and frequency of each marked symptom using the scoring system above. Where indicated, write in a number rather than using ticks. This goes in the No Appliance column if you do not use an appliance while sleeping and in the With Appliance column if you do.
- If you currently sleep using an appliance, go down the 'My Symptoms' list again and using a different coloured pen, record your ratings in the No Appliance column for how the symptoms were before you used an appliance. For example, with your oral splint in, you might only go to the toilet once a night now, but you may have previously been waking three times to go. (See example and explanation.) There may also be some other symptoms in the list that you used to have before you got your device. These also need to be identified with an X and rated in the No Appliance column, using that different coloured pen. For instance, previously you may have snored heavily all night but now on CPAP you do not snore. (See example.)
- Symptom Score = total of numbers + ticks.
  Add up the number of ticks, plus the value of the numbers in the No Appliance and With Appliance columns, and record the result in the space at the bottom. This gives you a Symptom Score. If you are using an appliance, you will have two Symptom Scores – your current Symptom Score and another reflecting how things were before you used an appliance.

Opposite is an example of a Symptom Tracker for someone who snores and is currently wearing an oral splint. It shows how the person arrived at a current and prior Symptom Score. (It is usual to have more symptoms than shown in the example opposite.)

SYMPTOM TRACKER EXAMPLE

MY SYMPTOMS	SYMPTOMS	ASSESSMENT 1 Date:		ASSESSMENT 2 Date:	ASSESSMENT 3 Date:
		NO APPLIANCE	WITH APPLIANCE Type: Splint		
X	Snoring	✓ ✓ ✓			
X	Blocked or stuffy nose	✓ ✓	✓ ✓		
X	Waking self with snort (Average number per night)	3			
X	Toilet visits overnight (Average number per night)	3	1		
X	Sighing	✓ ✓ ✓	✓ ✓ ✓		
	SYMPTOM SCORE TOTAL	14	6		

In the (abbreviated) example given, for a person using an oral splint, the subject:

- used to snore virtually all night long most nights; no snoring now they use oral splint.
- has a stuffy nose most mornings (no change).
- used to wake self with a snort three times most nights; now uses splint and does not wake with a snort.
- used to make three toilet visits overnight; now using splint, it is usually only once.
- sighs a lot throughout the day (no change).
- had a Symptom Score of 14 prior to oral splint; now using splint, score is 6.

TABLE 4.3: SYMPTOM TRACKER

MY SYMPTOMS	SYMPTOMS	ASSESSMENT 1 Date:		ASSESSMENT 2 Date:	ASSESSMENT 3 Date:
		NO APPLIANCE	WITH APPLIANCE Type:		
	Snoring				
	Irregular breathing during sleep				
	Restless/ interrupted sleep				
	Insomnia				
	Recalled wakings (Average number per night)				
	Waking self with gasp/snort (Average number per night)				
	Toilet visits overnight (Average number per night)				
	Frightening or vivid dreams				
	Shuddering in sleep, legs jerking or twitching in bed				
	Waking tired				
	Waking with a headache				
	Waking with dry mouth or throat				
	Blocked or stuffy nose				
	Runny nose (Number of tissues used per day)				
	Post-nasal drip				
	Heavy or laboured breathing				
	Breath holding in the day				
	Sighing or extra-deep breaths				
	Frequent yawning				
	Irritable cough				
	Throat clearing				
	Short of breath when resting				
	Short of breath when reading or talking				

MY SYMPTOMS	SYMPTOMS	ASSESSMENT 1 Date:		ASSESSMENT 2 Date:	ASSESSMENT 3 Date:
		NO APPLIANCE	WITH APPLIANCE Type:		
	Easily breathless with exertion				
	Erratic or faster heartbeats				
	Difficulty swallowing				
	Feeling revved up, jumpy, irritable				
	Anxiety, tension, apprehension				
	Panic attacks				
	Feeling 'spaced out' or confused				
	Dizziness, light-headedness				
	Tingling in limbs or face				
	Poor concentration or memory				
	Frequent or urgent urination				
	Heartburn/gastric reflux/gut upsets				
	Excessive sweating				
	Chest wall sore to touch				
	Achy or tense muscles				
	Muscle spasms, tremors, twitching				
	General tiredness or weakness				
	Chronic exhaustion				
	Sleepiness during day				
	Falling asleep sitting, reading, watching TV, in a car				
	Needing and taking a day nap (Number of days per week)				
	SYMPTOM SCORE (ticks + numbers)				

√ = occasional

√√ = part of each day/night

√√√ = frequent, most of day/night

√√√√ = frequent and/or strong

Important note: This is not an exhaustive list of symptoms that can indicate dysfunctional breathing. Some symptoms of dysfunctional breathing or breathing pattern disorder mimic other more serious conditions; many of these symptoms may also be associated with other ailments and disorders. There may be a number of reasons for any particular symptom to occur and there may indeed be several different causes operating at once. Your doctor can determine this for you.

The breathing pattern and symptom self-assessment process used in this book is not intended to diagnose, and should not be taken as any kind of diagnosis of any disease or condition, including a diagnosis of breathing pattern disorder or sleep apnoea, or other sleep-breathing disorder. Nor is it a substitute for medical advice about any symptom or condition. While the self-assessment process in this book can give valuable information about your baseline breathing pattern and breathing habits, and may be very helpful in guiding you as to what you may be able change yourself to improve the way you breathe, it is not a substitute for medical diagnosis and advice.

If you have not already been medically diagnosed with sleep apnoea but suspect after reading Chapter 3 and doing this self-assessment process that you do have it, see your doctor, who can decide if your condition warrants investigation. Significant sleep apnoea is a very serious condition and needs to be addressed without delay.

Any health problem and any worrying symptoms, particularly anxiety, chest pain, chest tightness, shortness of breath, dizziness, tingling and breathing stoppages/apnoea should be checked by a doctor. Nonetheless, dysfunctional breathing – or more specifically, chronic over-breathing/ hyperventilation – is a well-documented contributory factor to the symptoms in this list.

KNOWLEDGE IS POWER

What we can say for certain is that if you have sleep apnoea or snoring, or both, your breathing-control mechanism is out of order. You have disordered breathing. You are definitely breathing incorrectly, and it won't be just at night.

But there's hope: when you know what is going on, you are in a better position to do something about it.

I hope the self-assessment procedures in this section have helped you to identify any areas where your breathing pattern falls short of normal. If it does, the symptoms you identified in Table 4.3 are likely to be connected with the way you breathe, and many of them may improve if you learn to breathe correctly. It is not your destiny to develop snoring or sleep apnoea just because, for example, 'it runs in the family'.

Awareness of these facts opens the way to a management approach – involving breathing retraining – that directly addresses faulty breathing habits. In my practice, I consistently see breathing retraining giving immediate relief and long-term benefits to people with breathing-related problems.

Breathing is retrainable. First you recognise your poor breathing habits, then you undo them, and then you get back to normal breathing and enjoy the benefits.

Stuart is a typical client. He is middle-aged, has had two lots of nasal surgery but came to me at his wife's urging as he was still snoring and both worrying and annoying her. Jane described Stuart's breathing at night: 'He breathes much faster than I do; sucks when he breathes in, and blows when he breathes out. I can't sleep when he is blowing a gale on my back!' All this wasn't bothering Stuart, but he was fed up with waking to go to the toilet, having a dry mouth and feeling really tired in the morning. (Jane added that he was becoming grumpy too.) The signs were there in the day as well – fast breathing, upper-chest breathing, lots of nose blowing and at least one sigh per minute.

Stuart was taught to use his diaphragm properly and how to slow down and get an even rhythm to his breathing. These changes helped to keep his nose clear. By the third night there was no snoring and both Stuart and Jane were waking refreshed.

CHAPTER 5

Normal, healthy breathing –
how do you measure up?

A big part of helping people breathe and sleep better comes when they really 'get it'. They get what they have been doing wrong breathing-wise, the likely reasons it happened, how it's led to their symptoms and what they can do about it right now. It's all very logical. No mystery, no leap of faith needed. To help you get it, I need to go into a little technical detail here about the ins and outs of breathing.

The main function of breathing is to bring about the exchange of oxygen and carbon dioxide and to maintain them at very particular levels for the optimal functioning of the body. They are both critical for life.

Oxygen makes up 20 per cent of the air you breathe in. You inhale it into your lungs, into the alveoli – the small air sacs where gases are exchanged. The oxygen then passes into your bloodstream. It attaches itself to the red blood cells (haemoglobin) and then is taken by the bloodstream to your organs and tissues. The haemoglobin then releases the oxygen, which moves into your cells, where it is used as fuel to 'burn' or oxidise fats and carbohydrates, making energy to drive your body. Fats and carbohydrates are mostly composed of carbon with some hydrogen and oxygen.

The main by-products of this energy production are carbon dioxide and water. The carbon dioxide moves out of the cells and into the blood. The bloodstream takes the carbon dioxide to your lungs where some (what is not needed) can be breathed out. Compared to what you breathe in, there is a lot more carbon dioxide in your blood, in your lungs, and in the air that you breathe out. Only a tiny amount (0.038 per cent) of the air you breathe in is carbon dioxide. Yet the ideal level of carbon dioxide to have in the air sacs in your lungs is 5.5–6.5 per cent.

Your body makes carbon dioxide and in effect concentrates it in your blood and lungs. You do not exhale to rid yourself of carbon dioxide, but to maintain it at the optimal level. Too much or too little is a problem. Therefore, breathing too much or too little is a problem.

WHAT DOES 'NORMAL' BREATHING LOOK LIKE?

A truly healthy person's breathing, whether they are awake or asleep, is easy; the rhythm is smooth and regular, with even timing and similar-sized breaths (see Figure 5.1, page 39). It is silent during the day and at night, silent with light activity, and even fairly quiet during moderate physical exercise. It is in and out through the nose, all day and all night and even with exercise. The breathing movement occurs predominantly at the diaphragm (solar plexus) level, and little if any movement of the upper chest, shoulder area and lower abdomen is seen.

The criteria of correct breathing are referred to as *physiological norms*. At rest, an adult should breathe eight to twelve times per minute. (A higher breathing rate is normal in children.) The volume of air inhaled and exhaled at each breath is called the *tidal volume*; the total volume of air breathed per minute is called the *minute volume*. The norm for tidal volume is 500 ml; 4–6 litres is the norm for minute volume.

You cannot accurately measure how much you breathe in during one breath or each minute yourself, and the equipment that measures this is usually only found in hospitals. However, you can get a fair indication by using the Sound and Airflow checks described earlier. An ideal-sized breath is silent and gives a sensation of warmth and a mere hint of airflow – an airflow rating of 1 or 2 as per the scale on page 24. (You're not embarrassed by the noise of your breathing when at the cinema, and will not get complaints from a bed partner about annoying noise and air gushing over them at night.)

At rest and during sleep, passing 4–6 litres of air per minute through your lungs supplies more than enough oxygen to load up (saturate) your haemoglobin with oxygen, and at the same time maintains the carbon dioxide level within the optimal range in your lungs and blood. During exercise, more carbon dioxide is produced and more oxygen is needed; a healthy breather naturally breathes faster and deeper during exercise. Less oxygen is needed during most stages of sleep, and the healthy breather naturally breathes less while asleep.

Now let's look at some of the features of healthy breathing more closely. First, the nose. The nose is well designed as a filter, heater, humidifier and cleaner of the air we breathe. It is quite capable of supplying enough air for a well-trained, healthy person to run a marathon.

The diaphragm also is perfectly designed for the job it is meant to do. This thin but powerful dome-shaped muscle is situated under your lungs, separating your chest cavity (containing lungs and heart) from your abdominal cavity (containing stomach, liver and intestines). It is the primary breathing muscle, and its action moves air in and out of the lungs. When your diaphragm contracts, the 'dome' flattens and pushes down on the upper-abdominal contents as the breath is drawn into the lungs.

With a normal-sized inhalation and diaphragm action, only a small outward (bulging) movement of the solar plexus area will be felt and be visible. The intercostal muscles (between the ribs) play a much more minor role in breathing. In quiet breathing your lower ribs flare out slightly to the side when you breathe in; the upper rib muscles remain relaxed. Minimal, if any, movement in the upper-chest area and lower abdomen is seen. Then the diaphragm relaxes, and the out-breath follows passively through the 'elastic' recoil of the lungs and diaphragm. Air flows silently from your lungs back through the upper airways into the atmosphere.

The diaphragm muscle adapts to your needs – it travels through a small distance when you are resting and sleeping; it will move through a greater distance to draw in more air when you are exercising.

HOW DO YOU COMPARE WITH NORMAL?

Compare the results from your assessments on pages 19 and 26 to the norms in Table 5.1 (page 39). (I suggest you write what is 'normal' down the right-hand sides of Tables 4.1 and 4.2, alongside each parameter.) If normal, healthy breathing is nasal, smooth, silent, small, soft, slow and relatively still, how do *you* compare?

If you are like the thousands of people with breathing-related problems who I have helped, you would have likely just established for yourself that you do not breathe correctly, either during the day or the night, and generally, or intermittently, breathe too much, particularly when you are asleep.

WHAT DOES POOR BREATHING LOOK LIKE?
Fast breathing

Poor breathers often, but not always, breathe faster than normal. The average respiration rate recorded for my adult clients (when awake) is sixteen breaths a minute, though rates up in the mid-twenties are not uncommon. This is significantly higher than the norm of eight to twelve. However, even rates over twenty breaths a minute may not be noticed by the person themself or a casual observer. I have counted rates over twenty in my fellow passengers snoring away on long-haul flights and train journeys.

Chest-breathing

Poor breathers are often chest-breathers (more precisely, upper-chest breathers) as opposed to diaphragm-breathers. They use the rib muscles and the accessory (shoulder and neck area) breathing muscles for a larger proportion of their breathing effort than does a healthy breather. Their upper chest moves before or more than their solar plexus and you may also see their shoulders and collarbones lifting. (Sometimes you see 'paradoxical' breathing, where the abdomen is actually drawn in on the in-breath.)

The accessory muscles are not meant to be so involved in normal resting breathing. They are muscles of 'desperation' rather than 'inspiration' – they are meant to be on standby for when increased lung capacity is needed, such as during intense exercise or in situations of fear or threat. The rest of the time breathing should be predominantly diaphragmatic – around 80 per cent of the breathing effort should be via the diaphragm, with the other 20 per cent supplied mainly by the rib muscles in the *lower* rib area. This means the upper chest should be virtually still.

Upper-chest breathing is far less efficient than diaphragm-breathing and seriously disadvantages you. These muscles tire easily and produce lactic acid, which is the reason many people wake up after a night of heavy snoring and erratic breathing with their chest feeling sore and bruised.

Irregular breathing

Irregularity in the breathing pattern is very common. Rather than the smooth, even pattern seen in healthy breathers, those who snore and suffer from sleep apnoea may have varying breath sizes and timing. During the day, breathing may be interrupted by yawning, sighing, throat clearing, extra-deep breaths, irritable coughing and breath holding.

During the night, there may be bouts of snoring, snorting, gasping and choking breaths, punctuated by periods of breath holding of varying lengths. Of course, there are accompanying sound effects as well. Conversely, with a healthy breather, you can be unaware they are sitting or sleeping beside you.

Mouth-breathing

Mouth-breathing during sleep is common in people with snoring and sleep apnoea. Mouth-breathing is a form of *over-breathing* (see below) – tidal volumes are invariably greater than normal and the air rushes in faster. The mouth after all is a much bigger opening than the sum of two nostrils. It's a well-known fact that both snoring and sleep apnoea are worse with mouth-breathing.

Over-breathing

Over-breathing is breathing more than normal – moving more air in and out of your lungs than is needed to fuel your current level of activity. If you are sleeping, or sitting reading this book, you only need around 5 litres of air each minute, which equates to about ten breaths of 500 ml each. Taking twenty breaths of 500 ml, or sixteen of 625 ml, will give you 10 litres of air consumption in a minute. This is significant over-breathing, but is likely to go unnoticed.

FIGURE 5.1: NORMAL BREATHING

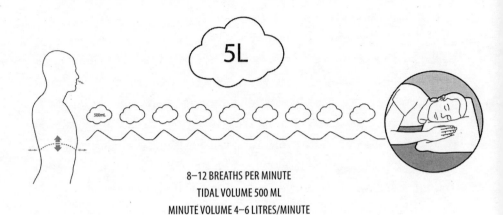

8–12 BREATHS PER MINUTE
TIDAL VOLUME 500 ML
MINUTE VOLUME 4–6 LITRES/MINUTE

TABLE 5.1: NORMAL BREATHING – AT REST

BREATHING PARAMETER	NORMAL CHARACTERISTICS/VALUES
Feel of breathing	Easy, satisfying
Rhythm	Regular, smooth
Sound	Silent
Respiration rate	8–12 breaths per minute
Route	Nose – rest, exercise, sleep
Location (dominant)	Diaphragm
Tidal volume	500 ml per breath (Airflow: 1–2)
Minute volume	4–6 litres per minute
Heart rate	60–80 beats per minute

Researchers have recorded average tidal volumes of 950 ml and average minute volumes of 15 litres/minute during the day, in men who have sleep apnoea.[5.1]

My observations of thousands of clients suggest that the majority of people with sleep-breathing disorders have excessive tidal volumes most of the time, even when they are nose-breathing. The evidence during the day is the heaviness of breathing, excess movement of the chest and abdomen, strong airstream from the nose or mouth, and audible airflow from the nose or mouth. Sometimes over-breathing is subtle and hard to detect. Breathing can be fast but not heavy or noisy; sometimes repetitive sighing or yawning is the only indication – but it is enough!

The tidal volume in sighs, yawns, gasps, coughs, snores and snorts is invariably larger than 500 ml. In fact, any noisy or 'drawn-out' breath is likely to be the same. Research suggests a typical sigh is around 1600–2000 ml and can be as high as 3000 ml – that's 3 litres! Some sighing is considered normal, but frequent sighing indicates a problem with breathing regulation. It is also a sign of anxiety and a body under stress.

Do you sigh a lot, clear your throat, or find yourself taking extra-deep breaths every so often? (Ask a work colleague or family member – they often notice this when you don't.) I've found sighing to be very common in people with sleep-breathing disorders – I have also seen it disappear very quickly through breathing retraining.

At night, over-breathing manifests as noisy, heavy and windy breathing, and the chest may heave. There is definitely not a normal tidal volume going in and out during snoring! To get an idea of just how excessive a snorer's breathing volume can be when compared to normal, think of it in terms of litres. It is normal to breathe around 5 litres of air per minute during sleep. Now for a heavy snorer who breathes 15 litres a minute, that's an extra 10 litres of air breathed every minute! Over an eight-hour night of heavy snoring that's an extra 4800 litres of air that the snorer breathes compared to the non-snorer. Can you imagine why the heavy snorer is going to wake up tired and with a dry mouth and sore throat?

During sleep, when the throat is relaxed, the high airflow rate creates turbulence and vibration in the back of the throat – and there you have it: the sounds of snoring. One woman I saw in my practice described her partner's tidal volumes: 'When he breathes in, it's like he is sucking the paint off the walls, and when he breathes out, I have to hold on in case he blows me out of bed.' Breathe in fast and heavily enough and you can actually suck your airway shut and stop breathing for a while.

Figure 5.2 shows you what disordered breathing looks like. The data in Table 5.2 (see page 42), estimated from surveying my clients at various times over a twenty-year period, gives you a picture of what is typical of people with breathing-related conditions.

FIGURE 5.2: DISORDERED BREATHING

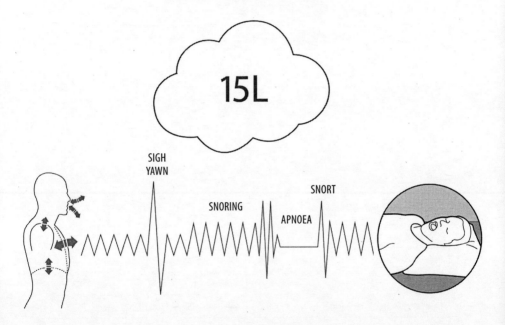

The bottom line is that your average snorer and apnoea sufferer has a dysfunctional breathing pattern. In other words, they breathe abnormally. The abnormality can be in any or all of the parameters discussed here, during the day and during sleep.

The most common and over-riding dysfunction I see in clients is over-breathing. Not everyone I have seen in my practice has been a mouth-breather, not everyone has been a fast breather or a chest-breather, not everyone has been constantly breathing heavily, but some signs of over-breathing have been present. People who snore or suffer from sleep apnoea are likely to either regularly or intermittently breathe enough air for two or three people.

Table 5.3 compares traits of a normal breather with those of an over-breather.

TABLE 5.2: TYPICAL BREATHING-CENTRE CLIENTS

Average respiration rate – 16 breaths per minute (range 6–28)
20% mouth-breathe all day
50% mouth-breathe part of the day
80% mouth-breathe at least at times during sleep
40% have audible breathing when awake
95% have audible breathing at least at times when asleep
70% are chest breathers at least at times
70% sigh or yawn excessively

TABLE 5.3: NORMAL BREATHING PATTERN VS OVER-BREATHING PATTERN

Normal breathing indicators	Typical over-breathing indicators
Regular, smooth	Irregular, sighs, yawns, coughs, snores, snorts
Silent	Audible, noisy
Eight to twelve breaths per minute	Over fourteen breaths per minute
Dominant diaphragm movement (small)	Obvious / large upper-chest movement and / or obvious abdominal movement
Nose-breathing	Mouth-breathing or 'heavy' nose-breathing
Gentle, soft breaths	High tidal volume, 'heavy', 'windy', full breaths

As well as considering the above indicators, you could stand in front of a mirror and observe your breathing. If the rise and fall of your chest is obvious, it is likely you are over-breathing.

The terms *hyperventilation* and *over-breathing* are generally interchangeable. However, I will mainly use the term *over-breathing* as most people connect hyperventilation with the obvious rapid breathing that occurs during a stressful event or with a panic attack. This 'acute' hyperventilation is easy to see, but chronic over-breathing is actually far more common, more subtle or 'hidden', and so often goes unrecognised. However, as I have explained, the indicators are there if you know what to look for. (Signs of over-breathing are also often observed in people with other breathing-related conditions including asthma, anxiety and panic disorders, COPD, frequent upper-respiratory infection, hayfever, chronic rhinitis and sinusitis.)

> **NOSE, MOUTH, SIGH – VOLUME COMPARISON**
>
> To compare the tidal volume of air used for nose- and mouth-breathing and when you sigh, try the following:
>
> 1. Place one hand on the upper chest and the other on the solar plexus. Note where and how much movement you feel when you nose-breathe.
> 2. Keeping your hands in place, now open your mouth and breathe through it. Did you notice an increase in the amount of movement, indicating a larger tidal volume?
> 3. Keep your hands in place and now sigh. Did you feel the upper chest heave?

Anyone who has slept downwind of a heavy snorer will identify with the concept of excessive breathing volume. It is no wonder snorers are more tired when they wake up than when they go to sleep. Their legs may have had a fair workout too. Or as the wife of one of my clients told me, 'You would think my husband was running a marathon all night, what with the threshing legs, heavy breathing and gasping.'

Does all this surprise you? Were you under the impression that breathing lots of air was good for you? This pervasive belief may well qualify as public-health enemy number one.

WHY IS OVER-BREATHING BAD FOR YOU?

Having the odd breath here and there out of balance is not a problem. But when most of the 20 000–25 000 breaths you take in a day are dysfunctional, the cumulative effect on your body's ability to function is significant. And in the same way you would expect consistent high blood-sugar levels, high blood pressure or a heart rate twice the norm to cause a problem or two, breathing at double or triple the normal rate also causes problems.

Chronic over-breathing is associated with a wide array of symptoms in any organ or system of the body, and can mimic serious disease. It has physical and mechanical effects on the tissues lining your nose, sinuses, throat and lungs; it alters normal blood chemistry; it has psychological effects; it has repercussions on the respiratory, cardiovascular, neurological, gastrointestinal and musculoskeletal systems. Over-breathing often holds the explanation for a wide range of health problems.

Are you starting to see how over-breathing could be behind many of the symptoms you have been suffering? In the next chapter we will explore this idea. But rest assured, there is a way out of this – you can change the way you breathe. In fact, changing poor breathing habits can be a lot easier than giving up some other habits – smoking, for example. Your body can begin to function again the way it was meant to, and it usually doesn't take long before you feel better.

> Glenda had been snoring heavily for over twenty years. Her husband Dave phoned to make an appointment for her and asked a few questions. After he realised that mouth-breathing was a problem (Glenda was a full-time mouth-breather), he encouraged her to breathe through her nose a little bit more each day. When Glenda came in for her appointment four days later she was able to report that she was snoring much less already – her snoring was now only intermittent, as well as considerably quieter. Also, she wasn't waking up so stiff in the legs, and she was waking up earlier and feeling more alert. Already she had much more energy. All Glenda had done was to try to keep her mouth shut during the day!

CHAPTER 6

The over-breathing model: A new way of looking at snoring and sleep apnoea

On first hearing the idea that over-breathing is a core factor in snoring and sleep apnoea, some people ask how this is relevant to them. They may have placed the blame on the shape of their jaw, the size of their tongue or the layer of fat around their neck. Or they may believe they are a hopeless case because their nose is always blocked, even after having surgery. Well, please hear me out.

While the presence of anatomical 'defects' may well compound the problem, over-breathing is still likely to be relevant to incidences of snoring and sleep apnoea. To understand this you need to look closely at what actually happens in your airway and in your body while you are breathing the way you do.

Despite considerable research over the last 30 years, there is still no clear consensus in the medical literature on the underlying cause of sleep-disordered breathing. However, certain risk factors for snoring and obstructive sleep apnoea have been identified. These include:
- being middle-aged
- being male
- being overweight or obese
- having particular anatomical features – large neck, recessed chin, narrow jaw, large tongue
- having large tonsils, adenoids or uvula
- nasal congestion or blockage.

WHAT'S WRONG WITH MOUTH-BREATHING?

Mouth-breathing may contribute to:
- bad breath, dental decay, gum disease
- dysfunction of the jaw joint (TMJ)
- narrowing of the dental arch, jaw and palate
- crowded and crooked teeth
- open bite, malocclusion (teeth not fitting together properly)
- greater potential for relapse of orthodontic corrections
- dysfunction of the muscles around the jaw and lips
- loss of lip tone, with the lips becoming flaccid
- noisy eating, speech and swallowing problems
- trauma to soft tissues in the airways
- enlarged tonsils and adenoids
- introducing unfiltered, poorly humidified air into the lungs
- upper-chest breathing (inefficient, tiring)
- chronic over-breathing
- greater incidence of snoring and sleep apnoea.

The last three points relate to the size of the space we breathe through. The narrower the upper-airway passage, the more likely it is that there will be air turbulence, soft-tissue vibration, snoring, and obstruction to the flow of air into the lungs. There are, however, some conundrums that the medical model of snoring and sleep apnoea cannot explain. Snoring and apnoea can occur without any of these predisposing or risk factors being present. A slim woman with healthy lungs and normal facial anatomy can develop sleep apnoea. Obstructive sleep apnoea can affect men, women and children of all ages and body types.

If we were to gather a roomful of people who have sleep apnoea, only some would be overweight, over 40, or have a deviated septum, stuffy nose, floppy uvula, recessed chin or a fat neck. However, the one factor that they would all have in common, I believe, is a *disordered breathing pattern*.

I also propose dysfunctional breathing as the menace behind many associated symptoms, such as nasal congestion, dry mouth, swollen adenoids and twitching legs – and even a narrow upper palate. Before blaming these things on pollens, your age or your genes, consider the role your poor breathing habits may play.

OVER-BREATHING AND SLEEP-DISORDERED BREATHING

The *over-breathing model* proposed in this book identifies over-breathing as a fundamental factor capable of precipitating a cascade of effects associated with sleep-disordered breathing. The explanations given here are kept as simple as possible. Those wanting to explore the science and research further can look to the texts and journal articles listed in the Chapter reference and resource material, page 225.

Airway narrowing

Narrow upper-airway passages, in one or several places between your nostrils and your trachea (windpipe) are a definite risk factor for snoring, upper airway resistance syndrome and obstructive sleep apnoea. The narrowing can be due to congestion and inflammation of the nasal, sinus or throat tissues. It can be a 'structural narrowing' due, for example, to a narrow upper jaw. There could be a combination of factors. What is the connection with over-breathing? Well, over-breathing plays a part in both airway inflammation and structural narrowing.

INFLAMMATION AND SWELLING – STUFFY NOSE, POLYPS, SWOLLEN THROAT

Excessive breathing such as heavy breathing, mouth-breathing and snoring can traumatise your airways. The tissues lining your nose, sinuses, throat and lungs can become dehydrated, inflamed and produce mucous. They can become swollen – fluid congestion (oedema) of mucous membranes is known to be a response to low carbon dioxide induced through over-breathing.[6.1] Mast cells in mucous membranes leak histamine – an inflammatory chemical – in response to low

NOSE-BREATHING MATTERS

Nose-breathing is beneficial because it:
- warms, moistens and filters the air.
- traps large particles with the nose hairs; small particles via mucous membranes.
- produces nitric oxide – a steriliser and bronchodilator.
- helps prevent colds, flu, allergy reaction, hayfever, irritable coughing.
- retains some moisture from exhaled air, preventing nasal dryness.
- provides a sense of smell.
- regulates (slows) airflow because of the nose's intricate structures.
- facilitates correct diaphragm action.
- promotes the parasympathetic nervous system, which calms and relaxes the body, slows the breathing and the heart, promotes digestion.
- allows the correct position of the tongue (against upper palate) and lips (together), assisting formation of the natural dental arches and straight teeth.
- reduces likelihood of snoring and apnoea.

carbon dioxide. Conversely, carbon dioxide stabilises mast cells, preventing histamine release.[6.2]

The result of over-breathing then can be a blocked, stuffy or runny nose, excess mucous, post-nasal drip, the growth of nasal or sinus polyps, and narrowed, congested and painful sinus passages. In the pharynx there may be reddening, swelling and enlargement of the uvula, the tonsils and the adenoids. Sometimes the tonsils and adenoids become so enlarged as to virtually block the airway, and this can be life-threatening.

STRUCTURAL NARROWING – CHANGING THE SHAPE OF YOUR FACE

Mouth-breathing can also narrow your upper airway through changing the shape of your face. With mouth-breathing, the tongue drops to the bottom of the mouth and often sits against the teeth, and the cheek muscles push inwards. The result is unnatural constrictive forces on the underlying bone structures.

The tongue does not sit in its optimal position at the roof of the mouth against the hard palate, where it provides the significant upward pressure that assists the midface and upper jaw to develop correctly.

When mouth-breathing has persisted since childhood the result can be underdevelopment of the upper jaw and a narrow, high-arched, V-shaped upper palate and dental arch. This narrows the airway space. As the width of the nose follows the width of the jaw, a narrow nose with narrow nasal passages may also be seen. Such structural narrowing of the jaw and upper airway passages predisposes you to snoring and sleep apnoea.

REDUCE OVER-BREATHING, REDUCE AIRWAY TRAUMA, REDUCE SNORING

If you can recondition your breathing and become more comfortable with nose-breathing, slower breathing and the correct amount of air (less), then you are reducing the irritation and trauma to your nasal tissues, adenoids, tonsils and the uvula. These tissues have the potential to heal. Even polyps can shrink. With less inflammation, there is more space to breathe through. In addition, with reduced breathing volume you require less space anyway.

Restoring nose-breathing is usually the first thing breathing retraining addresses. Now don't despair, even if you have not breathed through your nose for several decades. In the last twenty years I have observed many such cases who have come out the other side of the retraining process completely reformed.

Over-breathing and snoring

When someone with normal breathing is asleep, their breathing volume decreases. They are quiet and relatively still. However, with a snorer, an observer can see, hear and feel an increase in breathing volume, breathing rate or both. With loud snoring it is possible to be breathing even more air than a healthy breather does when they are exercising!

THE FASTER AND BIGGER YOU BREATHE, THE MORE YOU SNORE

The snoring noise is produced by high-speed breathing creating turbulent airflow as it passes through the soft-walled tube of the upper airway, vibrating the 'soft tissues' there. These include the soft palate, the uvula, the walls of the pharynx, the adenoids and tonsils, and the base of the tongue.

The narrower the passage and the higher the airflow rate, the greater the turbulence and vibration can be. This is called *the Venturi effect*. A good analogy is a river as it is entering a narrow gorge – the speed of the water flow increases and there is more turbulence and noise. When it rains heavily (an increased volume of water) the effect is even stronger. For you, a stressful day and digesting a big meal eaten just before bed will up the volume of air entering your throat, creating more turbulence, and you will snore more intensely.

You have to suck in a lot of air to maintain a good snore. Your airway won't rattle, vibrate and 'snore' if you breathe the normal 500 ml tidal volume slowly through your nose. However, you can create the snoring noise yourself on demand, as actors do in movies. Try it now by quickly sucking in a large breath through your mouth. Now try doing it breathing slowly and gently. Again, the most critical factor is the airflow rate: the millilitres per second.

Snoring is obviously linked to big breathing – you can feel it, hear it, even see it! What do you think might happen if you retrained your breathing-control centre and turned the dial down a bit?

FIGURE 6.1: RESETTING YOUR DRIVE TO BREATHE

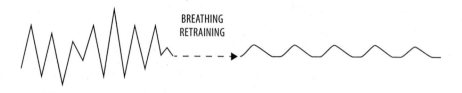

BREATHING
RETRAINING

Over-breathing, airway collapse and obstructive apnoea

Your airway narrowing or obstruction may have been attributed to a deviated septum, a large or floppy uvula, a small, receding jaw, or an overly large tongue falling backwards and blocking your airway. Anatomical features like these can certainly predispose you to snoring and obstructive sleep apnoea. So where does the over-breathing paradigm fit here?

If these anatomical features have been there longer than the snoring and apnoea have, and if your snoring and sleep apnoea are variable, there must also be a physiological (functional) factor involved besides the anatomical (structural) ones.

For example, you may have had a deviated septum and small jaw all your adult life, but the apnoea only started at age 45 and in the beginning at least was only happening some nights. You need to ask, has your breathing rate increased in this time? Has your partner complained in recent years how noisy your breathing is at the movies? Have you noticed your breathing is heavier than that of others at work or the gym? Has your dentist commented on the poor state of your gums – attributing it to mouth-breathing? Have friends commented on your sighing?

> Les realised his breathing had changed. He had been married for 30 years, and for the last few years, his wife had been forever telling him how noisy he was when sitting beside her, watching television. She also accused him of blowing air over her back while he was asleep.

When does sleep apnoea commonly occur? It is straight after a bout of big breathing or heavy snoring, or even after just one or two extra quick, large intakes of breath.

THE FASTER YOU BREATHE, THE GREATER THE SUCTION

The speed at which you inhale is called your *inspiratory airflow rate*. It reflects the set point of the breathing-control centre in your brain. People who chronically over-breathe have a higher drive to breathe, and a higher than normal airflow rate. There is research showing faster airflow rates in men with obstructive sleep apnoea than those without the condition.[6.3] Now, the faster the flow of air through the airway, the greater the *negative pressure* – vacuum or suction force – created on the walls of the passage (*the Bernoulli effect*). In other words, the airway walls move closer to each other the faster you breathe.

When you add chaotic, extra-large and fast intakes of breath, like snores and snorts, to an already high air-intake rate, and couple it with the more relaxed state of the throat 'dilator' muscles during sleep, it may create a suction effect sufficient to narrow or collapse the airway, partially or completely obstructing the airflow to the lungs. (There is also potential for the abnormal pressure changes in the throat to suck up acid from the stomach, further irritating the upper airways. Acid reflux or heartburn is a reasonably common accompaniment to sleep-disordered breathing.)

Imagine sucking so hard and fast on a paper straw in a milkshake, that the straw collapses, stopping the flow. Sucking harder would only make it worse. But if you worked the straw back into shape, and then tried sucking again more gently and slowly (lower flow rate – lesser volume of milk per second), the straw wouldn't collapse and you'd be able to finish your drink. Likewise, if you train yourself to breathe less air per second, you may well prevent your throat from collapsing.

THE ROLE OF THE DILATOR MUSCLES

The dilator muscles in the throat contract as you breathe in. Normally they maintain adequate 'tone' to counteract the suction pressure on the walls of the pharynx, to keep your throat open. During sleep general muscle tone decreases, including that of the throat dilators, and it is normal for the airway to narrow slightly and potentially have some increased resistance to airflow.

However, this is balanced by the natural reduction in tidal volume in healthy people during sleep. Therefore, while the upper airway is potentially more prone to collapse during sleep, there should be at the same time less suction applied to it. So, in normal circumstances, less dilator muscle activity is needed to maintain an open airway. Our airways are, in fact, inherently stable – the human body really is amazingly well designed. But we can muck it up by breathing too much.

Both snoring and apnoea tend to be worse with mouth-breathing and sleeping on your back. Big breathing is a culprit again as both habits increase tidal volume. In addition, gravity comes into play when you lie on your back. Your uvula, tongue and lower jaw are more likely to drop backwards. The over-breathing model also explains why your snoring and apnoea are worse when you are more stressed or when you eat a big meal close to bedtime. You breathe more in each of these circumstances, as you also do when you have a cold or if you are overweight.

Ultimately, the volume of air you breathe per second is a core factor in whether you will snore or not, and the chance of your throat collapsing. A selection of additional scientific literature relevant to this discussion is provided in Chapter references 6.4–6.10 (see page 227).

Please note: the implication of over-breathing in many instances of snoring and sleep apnoea does not discount cases where surgery or use of an oral device or positive air pressure is essential to maintaining an adequate airway space, where, for example, due to a structural problem, the airway physically 'over-closes' when the person lies down.

Over-breathing and central sleep apnoea

Let us consider for a moment how the over-breathing model fits with central sleep apnoea. In central sleep apnoea, breathing stops when the brain's breathing-control mechanism – the respiratory centre – fails to send a message to the diaphragm to contract and initiate breathing.

The breathing reflex is triggered according to the level of carbon dioxide in the arterial blood. If the level drops below a critical point, as it can do through over-breathing, the breathing reflex is depressed and breathing stops. The carbon dioxide level at which this happens is called the *apnoeic threshold*. Once breathing has stopped, the carbon dioxide level in the blood starts to climb. Once it reaches a certain point, breathing is stimulated again – the diaphragm contracts, the breath is taken, and air flows once more.

People with central apnoea do not always snore. However, research has certainly identified over-breathing in central sleep apnoea sufferers and linked it with the apnoea. Breathing volumes up to 20 litres per minute have been recorded in the phases before apnoeas occur.

Carbon dioxide is so vital to the ways our bodies function that we are all sensitive to any change in its level. In someone with central sleep apnoea, the apnoeic threshold may be just below their usual baseline carbon dioxide level, and just two or three brief dips (two or three extra-big breaths) can be enough to induce central apnoea. Conversely, preventing hyperventilation and keeping the carbon dioxide level above the person's threshold can prevent apnoea occurring. Research also shows carbon dioxide levels are relevant in obstructive sleep apnoea. (Chapter references 6.11–6.18 relate to this discussion, see pages 227–28.)

Life cannot be sustained if carbon dioxide drops too low, so at times central apnoea could actually be seen as a life-saving defensive mechanism. Put another way, apnoea could be seen as a response to the problem – the problem of breathing too much.

With mixed sleep apnoea it seems that sometimes the airway obstructs first; other times it's the drop in carbon dioxide that stops the breathing. If breathing doesn't stop completely, the body's compensation for over-breathing can be a period of significantly reduced airflow – hypopnoea. Again we see over-breathing as the likely common thread.

How breathing starts again (then stops again)

During apnoea, arterial blood oxygen drops and carbon dioxide starts to climb. The brain will wake the sleeper to kick-start breathing again. There is arousal, the dilator muscles of the pharynx are activated, the throat opens and breathing restarts. However, after this process, the breathing is dysfunctional. The next breath is usually an extra-large, quick gasp or snort. (These particularly large – and particularly loud – breaths are what partners notice.)

And then what do you suppose might happen? The next apnoea or hypopnoea can be triggered within a few breaths. The throat may narrow or collapse due to the vacuum effect, and/or the carbon dioxide can drop below the apnoeic threshold. And so on, the cycle repeats, again and again throughout the night.

These natural physiological mechanisms also explain why some people with sleep apnoea notice themselves holding their breath at times during the day. The breath-holds can be a response to, or compensation for, the big carbon dioxide-dumping sighs they are prone to. I call this 'day apnoea' and it's quite logical. Obviously if your breathing regulator is driving you to breathe erratically – 15–20 litres per minute at night – it is unlikely you will wake up and breathe a smooth, regular 5 litres per minute during the day!

Intermittent over-breathing

Not everyone who snores and/or has sleep apnoea is over-breathing all the time. Some appear to have fairly normal tidal volumes most of the day but will have intermittent big breaths or bouts of over-breathing particularly when they're stressed and chest-breathing. Variable or unstable breathing is another marker of a breathing pattern disorder.

Over-breathing and biochemical imbalance

We manufacture carbon dioxide from metabolism and physical exercise and store it in our lungs and blood. If you consistently over-breathe or hyperventilate, the amount of carbon dioxide in your body will fall below the optimal level, disturbing and destabilising body chemistry. Let us now consider the biochemical consequences of over-breathing and how they fit in with symptoms and conditions commonly seen in people with sleep-disordered breathing.

THE IMPORTANT ROLES OF CARBON DIOXIDE

Far from being a waste gas, carbon dioxide has many important roles as a regulator of body functions and processes. When it drops too low there are serious repercussions. We have already seen how a drop in carbon dioxide can trigger central sleep apnoea and release histamine into your airways.

One of carbon dioxide's most vital roles is ensuring cells take up oxygen. During normal breathing, your oxygen carriers, the haemoglobin molecules in your red blood cells, have nearly maximum oxygen saturation. That is, they are already fully loaded up with oxygen. Therefore, bigger breaths do not increase available oxygen. In fact, haemoglobin molecules must release their oxygen payload for it to be available to the cells, and carbon dioxide is needed for that to happen. The more carbon dioxide in the blood, the more oxygen gets released from haemoglobin, and the more cells are oxygenated (this is called *the Bohr effect*).

The other side of the equation is that when carbon dioxide is too low, the bond between the haemoglobin and oxygen tightens. Oxygen clings to the red blood cells, less is released, and cells can become starved of oxygen. With over-breathing, even though oxygen is plentiful in the blood, less of it is available to the cells. So the deeper and faster you breathe, the more carbon dioxide you blow off, and the less oxygen your tissues and vital organs get. You become *hypoxic* – low in oxygen.

**CARBON DIOXIDE –
NOT JUST A WASTE GAS**

Carbon dioxide:
- is the body's natural bronchodilator, antihistamine, tranquilliser and muscle relaxant.
- assists blood flow and oxygen transport by relaxing blood vessels.
- facilitates oxygen delivery to cells by displacing oxygen from the haemoglobin.
- enhances digestion by relaxing the walls of the gut.
- regulates activity of the nervous system.
- balances and regulates pH (acid–alkaline balance).
- plays an important role in electrolyte balance and metabolism.
- plays an important role in synthesis and regulation of antibodies, hormones and enzymes.
- regulates the rate and depth of your breathing.
- confers efficiency and stability to breathing when maintained in the normal range.

Have you ever felt dizzy or light-headed after taking deep breaths or blowing up a balloon too quickly? The brain and heart are such heavy users of oxygen that the deleterious effects of over-breathing are often noticed there first. Over-breathing can reduce oxygen supply to the brain by as much as 40 per cent, making it difficult to concentrate. It is common for over-breathers to often feel 'spaced out'.

When the oxygen supply to muscles is poor, cells can switch to *anaerobic* metabolism – energy production without oxygen. Lactic acid builds up in your muscles to give you that achy, tired feeling. After a night of over-breathing, some people wake up feeling like they've been pushing a truck uphill. Generally it is the legs where it's noticed, though I've had clients who talk about aching all over. The aching can also be experienced in the chest muscles, which are not designed for continual use.

Another vital role of carbon dioxide is that it regulates the acid–alkali (pH) balance in your body. There is an optimal and quite narrow pH range in which our body chemistry functions best. Therefore a chronic deficiency of carbon dioxide can compromise many body processes.

For years now, every morning George had woken up feeling like he had run a marathon – every part of his body, every muscle was aching and sore to the touch. After three days of breathing training, George declared that he was sleeping better and his mouth wasn't dry in the morning. But the most amazing thing for him was that he wasn't aching when he woke up.

Carbon dioxide has a calming and stabilising effect on nerve cells, and sleep comes more easily with a relaxed nervous system. When carbon dioxide is low, the nervous system becomes agitated. The (sympathetic) fight-or-flight response is turned on, you are on red alert, and your rest-and-digest (parasympathetic) system is short-changed. You may experience nervousness, anxiety, over-excitability, insomnia, general muscle tension and muscle twitches, and may even wake up covered in sweat.

Muscles, as well as nerves, are affected by low carbon dioxide. The smooth muscle lining of your airways, blood vessels, gut and bladder (and the uterus in women) can spasm and constrict. Headaches, asthma, shortness of breath, difficulty swallowing, high blood pressure, palpitations, poor circulation, heartburn, stomach cramps, colic, irritable bowel, menstrual cramps and urinary frequency and urgency are just some of the possible consequences of smooth muscle spasm and dysfunction. Blow off your carbon dioxide at your peril!

> Terry had recurring chest pain. A stress test performed by his cardiologist did not show any problem with blood flow to his heart. Terry was then referred to me. At his first appointment I could hear him breathing while he was still in reception. I counted his respirations at seventeen breaths a minute coupled with upper-chest breathing and a slumped posture. From the first day of retraining, Terry began to improve his breathing mechanics and reduce his over-breathing pattern. The chest pains resolved after the first session.

Carbon dioxide also has its crucial role in breathing regulation. The respiratory centre in the brain regulates the rate and depth of your breathing by the amount of carbon dioxide in your arterial blood.

OVER-BREATHING – OVER-LOOKED

You may be wondering why you haven't heard about the role the *way* you breathe plays in snoring and sleep apnoea until now. I believe there are several reasons for this. First, screening for a dysfunctional breathing pattern is not part of standard medical diagnosis. Second, the focus in treatment of snoring and sleep apnoea appears to be on the particular tissues that vibrate, narrow the airway, or obstruct airflow, more so than on the actual manner of breathing. Last, it seems that today we can be so disconnected from our bodies and so taken in by technology that we do not think to look closely at ourselves for either the source of a problem or its solution. Many people don't even see snoring as to do with breathing!

SUMMING UP

While there is considerable variation in people's breathing patterns, in my experience, disturbed breathing rhythm and chronic or intermittent over-breathing are characteristic of people with snoring and sleep apnoea.

The more you over-breathe:

- the greater the trauma, inflammation and swelling of tissues in the nose and throat.
- the greater the vibration and turbulence in your upper airway.
- the louder you snore.
- the lower the carbon dioxide level in the lungs.
- the greater the suction effect on your airway.
- the greater the tendency of your airway to collapse (OSA).
- the closer you get to the apnoeic threshold at which breathing may cease (central sleep apnoea).
- the more effects you may experience from disturbed breathing regulation, altered blood chemistry and impaired oxygenation; for example, anxiety or other psychological effects, or respiratory, cardiovascular, neurological, gastrointestinal or musculoskeletal symptoms.

A natural and logical way to avoid this cascade of effects is to retrain your breathing pattern to the correct rate, volume, mode and rhythm, which is eight to twelve breaths per minute, 4–6 litres per minute, nose-only breathing, gentle diaphragm-breathing and silent, regular, even breathing. You *can* learn to breathe again the way you did before you started snoring. You can reset your 'drive to breathe'.

FIGURE 6.2 : THE OVER-BREATHING MODEL

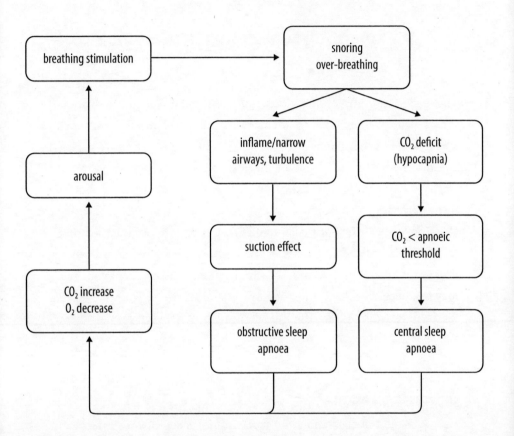

CHAPTER 7

Explaining those other symptoms

The over-breathing model does not contradict current mainstream theories, but rather adds to them and neatly explains inconsistencies and anomalies that confound them. This model also elegantly explains common symptoms associated with sleep-disordered breathing.

A loss of carbon dioxide from the body through over-breathing means arteries constrict, blood flow reduces, and the body is unable to absorb oxygen in the optimal amounts required to support all the important and interrelated functions of the body. Genetic predispositions are important factors in determining which systems or organs of your body may be affected.

Here we will look in more detail at the link between over-breathing and a few of the common symptoms and conditions associated with sleep-disordered breathing.

SHORTNESS OF BREATH
Shortness of breath frequently accompanies sleep-disordered breathing. As a sleep apnoea condition worsens, people may report increased breathlessness even when walking on flat ground. Breathlessness can occur on lying down, or you may wake with it. It can have various causes, including heart and lung diseases, but can also occur without any diagnosed disease. Breathlessness can be a consequence of poor breathing mechanics, excessive use of the inefficient chest muscles, or impaired oxygen uptake associated with an over-breathing pattern. Low carbon dioxide may trigger bronchospasm in susceptible people.

Some people who over-breathe say that they can 'never get enough air' no matter how deeply they breathe. Paradoxically, their breathing becomes more comfortable and they do not feel short of air when they learn to breathe less.

> Nine-year-old Jack was referred to me as he was breathless all the time and doctors could find no trace of asthma. A major clue was that he had been snoring for years and was a 100 per cent mouth-breather. With breathing retraining, Jack became a 100 per cent nose-breather within days, playing basketball without losing his breath and running faster than ever before.

FATIGUE, DAYTIME SLEEPINESS, POOR CONCENTRATION AND MEMORY

These symptoms are not just a result of disturbed sleep. They relate to being poorly oxygenated.

If you have simple snoring, or suffer from only mild apnoea, a sleep study would probably show that you have adequate oxygen saturation all night. However, 'brain fog', fatigue on waking, and low energy levels during the day suggest you *do* have an oxygen problem, even if it is not as obvious as it is for those with serious sleep apnoea.

Your over-breathing in the form of heavy snoring can mean that your oxygen intake and saturation remain high while the oxygen available to your tissues is compromised (*the Bohr effect*). Fatigue and other troublesome symptoms that people often put down to 'getting older' improve markedly or even disappear as soon as they rectify their breathing pattern.

HEADACHES

Headaches can have various causes, but one is certainly related to breathing. Headaches can occur in response to changes in the tone – constriction and dilation – of arteries feeding the brain. As you know by now, carbon dioxide affects the tone of the smooth muscle in arteries. Fluctuations in carbon dioxide with erratic breathing and apnoea may mean that you wake with a headache. Significant reduction in headaches is reported following breathing retraining.

NIGHT-TIME TOILET VISITS

Research shows an association between sleep-disordered breathing and night-time urination. When you over-breathe, the drop in blood carbon dioxide increases tension in smooth muscle, including that around the bladder. The increase in pressure on the bladder drives the need to urinate. In addition, there are shifts in pH and compensatory adjustments in electrolyte levels in the blood which increase urine production.

During the deep-sleep stages many of the hormones produced by your body for everyday life are made. One of these hormones is ADH (anti-diuretic hormone), which enables your body to concentrate urine. If you hyperventilate during sleep, you disturb the natural sleep cycles and spend less time in deep sleep, and so may find you need to pass urine more frequently. One of the first things many people notice when they improve their breathing is a reduction in daytime and night-time toilet trips (and in bedwetting in children).

> John came to the breathing class in the hope of putting an end to his snoring, which was driving his wife crazy. The snoring wasn't bothering him, but having to get up to go to the toilet three times a night certainly was. He thought there was something wrong with his bladder or, even worse, his prostate. John hadn't yet got around to doing anything about it, but three nights into the breathing course he started to sleep right through the night. He also noticed a reduction in frequency of daytime urination. John was happy, and so was his wife!

RESTLESS LEGS

This unpleasant creeping or crawling sensation in the legs generally occurs just before going to sleep. The sufferer will move their legs about to relieve the sense of unease. The discomfort and irritation can prevent sleep and contribute to daytime sleepiness. Another condition is 'periodic limb movement', where there is involuntary leg twitching or jerking during sleep. This can severely disrupt sleep, including that of your partner.

Your doctor may prescribe medications that may help the symptoms but are not curative.

Disturbed sensations and tremors in the limbs are also classic symptoms of hyperventilation. Low carbon dioxide can cause excessive activity in the nerves connecting to muscle, resulting in twitching and tremors. It's common for people to report the disappearance of these leg symptoms within 24 hours of commencing a breathing retraining program – even faster than conquering snoring, and that's saying something!

SEXUAL DYSFUNCTION

It's not just the annoyance of snoring and the debilitating fatigue occurring with sleep-breathing disorders that affects sexual relationships. Sexual arousal is controlled by the parasympathetic or relaxation part of your involuntary nervous system.

Over-breathing, on the other hand, heightens the sympathetic, or fight-or-flight, part of the nervous system. It is associated with stress responses including increased heart rate, blood pressure and blood supply to vital organs like the brain and lungs and away from low-priority tissues, which include the reproductive organs. (Reproduction is not a high priority when the body is under stress or threat.)

So if you are over-breathing, you can be in a state called 'sympathetic dominance', which will prevent proper activation of the parasympathetic responses during the arousal stage of sexual intimacy. It is no coincidence that erectile dysfunction is associated with sleep-disordered breathing.

INSOMNIA

Insomnia – difficulty falling asleep, staying asleep, or returning to sleep if awakened – is classified as a sleep disorder. It can be short-term, as with jet lag, when you first begin shift work or when you have a stressful event on your mind, or it can be chronic. Insomnia can be associated with pain and anxiety, with the use of some prescription and over-the-counter medications and with alcohol, caffeine and nicotine (cigarettes).

If insomnia occurs night after night it can be quite debilitating. It is estimated that up to 25 per cent of the population suffer from insomnia at some stage of their lives, and about 10 per cent have chronic insomnia.

If you have chronic insomnia you should discuss it with your doctor as it can occur in association with other illnesses, such as depression, anaemia and thyroid disease.

Is there a connection between insomnia and breathing? There certainly is. Over-breathing excites your brain and makes muscles tense and can therefore aggravate and even trigger insomnia.

Insomnia can respond well to the calming effects of controlled breathing. Remember, carbon dioxide is a natural tranquilliser and muscle relaxant. Having adequate levels is important in falling asleep and staying asleep. In healthy people, breathing naturally reduces during sleep and a small increase in blood carbon dioxide level is normal. Then breathing naturally deepens towards morning and the drop in carbon dioxide is part of the mechanism of waking up. Chapter references 7.1–7.3 provide background reading (page 228).

You may be wondering how your breathing got off track in the first place. I will take you through a few of the reasons in the next chapter.

CHAPTER 8

Why me? How disordered breathing starts

While breathing is largely automatic, it is also wide open to influence. It is affected by stress and emotions; by physical and environmental factors including posture, diet, medications and breathing techniques you may have practised – for example, in sport training, yoga, Pilates, singing lessons or with a breathing teacher.

Poor breathing habits often develop over time without us realising. They can start very early – three-year-olds can snore, and from my observations around 50 per cent of primary school–aged children mouth-breathe. Let's have a look at some of the factors or situations that can contribute to the development of dysfunctional breathing.

- High stress levels and modern lifestyles play their role. Increased stress gets our brains firing and elevates our breathing and heart rate, and with a sedentary lifestyle this stimulation is not counterbalanced by physical activity. Workaholics, high achievers, people with big mortgages or financial problems, carers, students, victims of abuse, refugees, the anxious, the bereaved or workers made redundant, to name just a few, can potentially develop a stress-related breathing pattern disorder.
- The modern diet typified by the Standard American Diet (SAD), with its heavy bias towards processed foods and highly refined carbohydrates, does not supply the nutrients vital for optimal health; at the same time it can rev up your breathing rate via the blood sugar/adrenaline axis (see Chapter 22). Overeating and putting on a lot of weight can also increase your breathing rate.

- The hormonal fluctuations of the teenage years and women's menstrual cycles can affect breathing, as can the changes during pregnancy and menopause.
- Chronic pain and illness and any accompanying anxiety can elevate your breathing rate.
- Recurrent sinus infection, chronic cough, and chronic mouth-breathing will affect your breathing pattern.
- Having a job (or personality) that requires a lot of talking can be an issue.
- The oh-so-common slumped sitting posture of the office worker, the texting teenager and the television watcher is a major factor in the development of an upper-chest breathing habit.
- Over-heating while sleeping, from too many bedclothes or an overly warm bedroom, can provoke over-breathing.
- An 'over effort' to maintain a flat stomach or improve 'core stability' by consciously tensing the abdominal muscles interferes with the movement of the diaphragm and therefore your breathing – this may potentially induce an upper-chest breathing pattern.
- A long-term habit or practice of overly filling and forcefully emptying the lungs of air or even repeated episodes of long-duration intense physical exercise where breathing is strained may imprint a chronic over-breathing pattern.

Please note: An increased respiratory drive can also be caused by, or be part of the body's way of compensating for certain conditions such as anaemia, diabetes, renal acidosis, liver failure, COPD or morbid obesity. If you have any doubt about your particular situation check with your doctor. (Also see Important note, page xi.)

BAD HABITS, BAD BREATHING

Like any habit, poor breathing is formed through repetition. You can develop upper-chest breathing through persistent stress, poor posture and mouth-breathing. Some people develop the habit of taking large sharp intakes of air when they begin to speak, and at each breath thereafter.

If they have a job or personality whereby they talk a lot, then that's a lot of over-breathing.

Mouth-breathing may begin with a blocked nose due to a cold, but it can persist long after the cold and mucous have gone. Mouth-breathing can get to the stage where you are so used to all that extra air that you feel like you will suffocate if you go back to nose-breathing, despite your nose being clear.

In children, the open-mouth posture affects muscle tension around the mouth and jaw, detrimentally influencing the alignment of their teeth and the shape of their face as they grow. Keep up mouth-breathing long enough and it can become difficult to close the lips without strain. Even throat clearing can become an unconscious bad habit.

CIRCUMSTANCES THAT IF PROLONGED MAY CONTRIBUTE TO THE DEVELOPMENT OF HABITUALLY DISORDERED BREATHING

bad posture
over-stimulation
high stress levels
emotional stress/shock
chronic cough
mouth-breathing habit
chronic pain
exercise with poor breath control
chronic infection
prolonged bed rest
over-heating
chemicals in the environment
over-sleeping
high-starch/high-sugar diet
overeating
poor nutrition
high caffeine intake
'too-deep' breathing exercises
forced exhalation exercises
excessive crying (children)
excessive alcohol consumption.

It is natural for your breathing volume to increase when you exercise, when you are ill or under stress or threat. What is not natural is when breathing does not return to normal once the exercise, illness, stress or threat is over. Excessive or long-term stresses, be they emotional, environmental or physical, may keep your breathing rate/volume disproportionately high for prolonged periods, just as persistent mouth-breathing can.

If you 'practise' faulty breathing habits long enough, they'll stick with you. Why? Because with repetition your body adapts, and the set point of the brain's breathing-regulation mechanism changes.

WHO ALTERED MY SETTING?

Breathing is highly regulated, with various physiological and biochemical feedback loops in play. The role of the respiratory centre in the brainstem is to regulate your breathing, keeping the carbon dioxide concentration at the optimal level (set point) so that all body processes function well. It operates much like an autopilot and means you don't generally have to think about your breathing.

Now, if you develop poor breathing habits that involve over-breathing, and you keep them up long enough, you over-ride this delicate reflex. When depletion of carbon dioxide is maintained over a critical period of time, your respiratory centre adapts and resets itself there. This will continuously drive your breathing at a higher rate, maintaining a sub-optimal carbon dioxide level by day and by night. You will have inadvertently changed the set point of your breathing and your *respiratory drive*. In this way over-breathing becomes automatic and chronic. You will likely feel that you are breathing 'normally'.

You don't just suddenly 'get' snoring and sleep apnoea, as if you were catching a cold. Usually your breathing has deteriorated over several years. It might have progressed from audible breathing during sleep to occasional 'social' snoring in your twenties after a few drinks, through to mild intermittent snoring most nights in your 30s, then heavy chronic snoring in your 40s (with added work stress and family responsibilities).

If not addressed, this progression may lead to sleep apnoea by the age of 50.

Even before you receive an official diagnosis of sleep apnoea, an alert observer may have noticed that your daytime as well as night-time breathing has become faster, heavier, more audible.

Many people report that their current condition developed or became worse after a major life event such as a significant injury or illness, job loss, divorce or bereavement. Even a bad cold or flu could be the trigger for persistent disordered breathing, especially if you did a lot of mouth-breathing and coughing while ill.

Although her pneumonia resolved after treatment with antibiotics and steroids, Kathleen noticed that she never returned to her pre-pneumonia state of health: fatigue and breathing discomfort persisted. Three months after this illness, she still could not manage the walk from home to the local shops, something she used to do most days. With breathing retraining she was soon back to her normal walking routine.

How many items in the list on page 67 are relevant to you? How much emotional, environmental or physical stress have you been exposed to? Has it been consistent enough to affect your breathing pattern? Your 'tipping point' – the point at which you develop chronic symptoms – depends on your baseline health, how many stresses you take on, and how big they are. It's a bit like a rain barrel – when it's full, all it takes is just one more drop of rain to make it overflow.

CHAPTER 9

Different approaches to
snoring and sleep apnoea

You may have already heard of many of the approaches offered by the sleep-medicine establishment. Here we will discuss some of the more common ones in the context of the over-breathing model. This discussion may help you understand some of the successes, benefits, failures and difficulties you have experienced along your journey with a sleep-breathing problem.

This section gives a general overview of the different treatment and management options currently available for people with sleep-disordered breathing. It is not intended to be an in-depth analysis, nor a complete summary of all that is on offer. Technological advancements in this field are happening all the time and surgical techniques and skills are constantly developing.

CONSERVATIVE APPROACHES

For simple snoring (snoring uncomplicated by sleep apnoea) or a mild sleep apnoea problem, your doctor may suggest you try conservative and self-help approaches before resorting to more interventionist treatments. For example:

- quit smoking
- lose weight
- minimise alcohol intake
- avoid tranquillisers and sleeping pills
- avoid sleeping on your back; elevate the head end of the bed

- nose-breathe during sleep
- commence a breathing retraining program.

There are various products available to encourage side-sleeping and nose-breathing. For example, there are special pillows that help you stay on your side, and *chin straps* to support your mouth in the closed position. There are also prescription medications and nasal spray preparations (medicated, herbal and saline) to reduce nasal congestion.

Breathing retraining is about identifying a person's dysfunctional breathing habits and teaching them better breathing skills. It is a 'big picture' approach as it incorporates education about lifestyle factors and habits that affect general health, breathing and sleep quality, including physical activity, diet and sleep positioning. The breathing retraining approach will be covered in detail in Chapter 10.

SURGICAL AND APPLIANCE-BASED APPROACHES

Most treatments offered by the medical and dental professions for snoring, upper airway resistance syndrome and obstructive sleep apnoea aim to increase or maintain sufficient opening in the upper airway to allow for continuous, non-restricted breathing during sleep. Choice of treatment depends on the nature and severity of the problem, and the other health conditions that may be present.

Surgery for snoring and sleep apnoea

Surgery can both increase the size of the airway opening and reduce the tendency of tissues to vibrate (flutter), collapse and obstruct the airway. More than one procedure may be needed.

Your doctor may suggest surgery to the nose and sinuses where bone, cartilage or soft tissues impede airflow through the nasal and sinus passages. These obstructions can include inflamed mucous membranes, nasal and sinus polyps, and a deviated nasal septum. People will feel, breathe and sleep better if surgery makes nose-breathing possible and comfortable. Some people have surgery to remove swollen tonsils or adenoids, and there are various procedures that remove, reshape and stiffen the tissue at the back end of the soft palate – which includes the uvula – so that it cannot vibrate. The soft palate and uvula procedures are most commonly used for snoring, and may be recommended for some people with obstructive sleep apnoea.

While less commonly performed, there is also surgery to reduce the size of the tongue or to pull the base of it forward, thereby enlarging the airway opening and preventing obstruction. There are also surgeries to reconstruct and reposition the lower jaw so that it no longer recedes.

Success rates vary between the different procedures. Reduction in snoring following a surgical procedure may not always be permanent, and reduction in snoring does not necessarily eliminate apnoea.

To me, over-breathing explains surgery that is only partially success-ful, as well as any relapses. Post-surgery, the patients have a larger and/ or more rigid opening to breathe through, but a continuing pattern of high-speed, high-volume breathing still has the potential to create suffi-cient suction on the airway walls to narrow and collapse them at some point, and other parts of the airway can still vibrate (snore) when relaxed during sleep.

In addition, persistent over-breathing has the potential to cause further inflammation of soft tissues and restrict airflow once again. Polyps can, and do, grow back.

Certainly, those people I have seen who have had only partial or impermanent success from surgeries had obvious breathing pattern dysfunction. When they sat in the consultation room breathing audibly twenty-plus times a minute, I had little doubt that over-breathing was behind their continuing snoring and/or apnoea.

Oral appliances

Since the early 1990s, dental/oral appliance therapy has increasingly become an accepted treatment for simple snoring, upper airway resist-ance syndrome and mild to moderate obstructive sleep apnoea. Oral appliances may be suggested for people who cannot tolerate CPAP treat-ment or as an alternative to surgery. There are various designs of these mouthguard-like devices (also known as splints) that fit over the upper and lower teeth and are worn during sleep. They reposition the lower jaw and/or push the tongue further forward. This creates a larger airway opening and effectively braces it by putting the walls of the upper airway under tension, so that they are less likely to vibrate or be sucked into a position that narrows the throat. Some types of devices can be bought over the counter or via the internet, and others are custom-made and fitted by dentists or orthodontists. It is generally recommended that people have a sleep study to first determine if an oral appliance is the most appropriate treatment for them.

Different devices produce different results. If the use of these devices brings about a significant improvement in snoring and apnoea, then they offer a real advantage compared to continuous positive airway pressure (CPAP) treatment in terms of simplicity, ease of use, portability and tolerance. While, in comparison to CPAP, oral appliances are not as effective in reducing the number of apnoea and hypopnoea episodes, compliance rates are higher.

Reasons given for discontinuing use of an oral appliance include ineffectiveness, irritation to soft tissues of the mouth (ulcers, for example), tooth discomfort (they can move teeth), a change in the bite, jaw pain, facial muscle discomfort and headaches. Wearing them may cause a dry mouth or the opposite, a saliva build-up. These problems, however, may only be mild and temporary. If persistent, they can lead to non-compliance. Professionally prepared, custom-made appliances are generally more effective and better tolerated than over-the-counter versions.

While oral appliances maintain a bigger and more tense airway opening, they do nothing about correcting the average snorer's dysfunctional breathing pattern with a high demand for air. They do, however, make it easier for the air to get through to the lungs.

Continuous positive airway pressure appliances

A CPAP appliance is the most common treatment for sleep apnoea. The person wears a mask over the nose, or nose and mouth, which is attached via tubing to an electrically driven air-compressor machine that delivers pressurised air into the airways during sleep.

The correct pressure to prevent the throat collapsing during sleep and eliminate apnoea is determined in an overnight sleep study. Some appliances start with low pressure and slowly increase it to help you adjust. Heated humidifiers are recommended for use with CPAP. There are other positive pressure appliances available with variable or 'bi-level' pressure for the different phases of breathing.

HOW CPAP WORKS

CPAP works in two related ways:

1. The positive pressure effect

CPAP prevents collapse of the airway by exerting a mechanical bracing or air splint effect on the throat. The positive air pressure puts the walls of the airway under tension and counteracts the negative pressure vacuum effect created on the airway wall as you breathe in. The air pressure is adjusted so that it is just enough to prevent episodes of obstructive apnoea.

2. Reducing the minute volume

By default, CPAP reduces over-breathing tendencies. When you are forced to breathe against pressure, your breathing rate and volume will automatically reduce. Research (into central sleep apnoea) has shown less air per minute was breathed when using CPAP compared to when sleeping without it, and that this resulted in a higher carbon dioxide level in the body.[9.1, 9.2] Maintaining carbon dioxide above the apnoeic threshold prevents episodes of central apnoea occurring.

BENEFITS OF CPAP

People with obstructive sleep apnoea benefit from both the positive air pressure and the reduced volume effects of using CPAP. Their throats are less prone to collapse due to the mechanical bracing and because there is less suction force on it when breathing less air per second.

CPAP, in effect, smooths out the breathing pattern. Huge breaths and sharp increases in flow rate are prevented; so are the sharp drops in carbon dioxide that can trigger apnoea. You breathe less air per second and per minute and breathing is more regular. When used correctly,

CPAP is indeed a very effective treatment for sleep apnoea.

The benefits are quickly seen. Sleep quality and blood oxygen levels improve and there is less daytime sleepiness. Treatment with CPAP has also been found to reduce blood pressure and improve heart function in people with congestive heart failure. A major advantage of CPAP is that it does not involve surgery and therefore avoids surgery's risks and potential side-effects.

A downside, however, is that it has little if any carry-over effect in improving breathing. During the day, the person resumes their 'default' faulty breathing pattern, and many will need even stronger CPAP pressures over the years if the underlying breathing dysfunction worsens.

And herein lies a major problem – it's a well-established fact that CPAP compliance rates are very poor. Not surprisingly, many people find sleeping with a mask strapped to their face every night hard to tolerate. The use of CPAP on a nightly basis for the rest of your life can be a daunting prospect and many reject it.

TAKE-UP AND COMPLIANCE WITH CPAP TREATMENT

Estimates for non-use or non-adherence to treatment in those for whom CPAP is the recommended option can be greater than 50 per cent. An Australian report by the National Health and Medical Research Council in 2000 found that 'a little less than half (46.2 per cent) of the initial group of patients considered for nCPAP [nasal CPAP] used the treatment for more than one month'.[9.3] A more recent report from the USA cites adherence rates ranging from 30 to 60 per cent.[9.4]

The number of CPAP machines sold certainly is not an accurate reflection of the number in use. If the owner finds CPAP intolerable, they may sell the machine or stash it away in the shed. People who have discarded their CPAP are often reluctant to tell their doctor.

There are a number of complaints about CPAP therapy that relate to this non-compliance. Some people find it claustrophobic, cumbersome and uncomfortable; that it restricts their position in bed and is inconvenient with travel. There may be emotional, social and aesthetic objections to wearing a face mask and being attached to a machine at night. There can be difficulty adapting to the air pressure; there may also be abdominal bloating. Some people have problems related to mask discomfort or due to air leaking from an ill-fitting mask and causing sore dry eyes or disturbing their partner's sleep. Nasal congestion or nasal dryness may also be a problem.

Many people go to the extra expense of buying a humidifier, but that can come with its own set of problems. An increased tendency to colds may be blamed on the humidifier; and moisture build-up in the mask that needs to be emptied during the night paradoxically may end up repetitively disrupting sleep. I have on occasion heard from clients that they 'take the whole thing off to get some sleep'.

As a 'gold standard' treatment CPAP seems to have some major short-comings for many people.

CPAP – FEELINGS OF CLAUSTROPHOBIA, PANIC AND 'DROWNING' EXPLAINED

I believe a key reason a large number of people can not tolerate CPAP is that it may force them to reduce their breathing rate and volume and raise their carbon dioxide level too quickly; that is, before their blood and their brain have had time to adjust.

When you are forced to breathe through your nose against a positive air pressure, your breathing rate will automatically reduce, and the carbon dioxide level in your lungs and blood will rise immediately. Although you are now protected from both obstructive and central sleep apnoea, the respiratory centre in your brain has not had time to readjust to the new breathing rate and carbon dioxide level.

When you have been used to high-volume breathing in the form of repetitive sighing, mouth-breathing, snoring or breathing heavily or rapidly for years, the sudden change using CPAP can be very difficult to tolerate. Your breathing is reduced mechanically, but your brain still wants you to breathe at the higher rate. Concerns reported to me include feelings of panic, claustrophobia and even a feeling of drowning.

Breathing retraining gets around this problem by gradually, during the day, bringing breathing closer to a normal rate, rhythm and volume, allowing you to acclimatise slowly and comfortably to the changes.

For many people, breathing retraining makes CPAP more tolerable. It brings about a natural calming of breathing that allows a better 'fit' between how much the person wants to breathe and what the CPAP machine allows them to breathe.

It's time to take a closer look at the breathing retraining approach.

CHAPTER 10

The breathing retraining approach

The options for treating snoring and sleep apnoea I've discussed in the previous chapter do not provide the whole answer. There is another approach, one that is conservative, science-based, natural, and gets back to first principles.

In this chapter, I look at the *breathing retraining approach* for people with sleep-disordered breathing.

KEY CONCEPTS
Faulty breathing patterns are characteristic of sleep-breathing disorders
If you have sleep apnoea and/or snore, then you have a disordered breathing pattern. No question. Though generally more obvious during sleep, the signs are usually also present when awake – such as upper-chest breathing, mouth-breathing, sighing, heavy, irregular and fast breathing, or gasping inhales during speech.

Snoring and sleep apnoea are fundamentally breathing problems
These common conditions are directly related to abnormality in the breathing function but may be perceived and treated only as anatomical or mechanical problems, needing surgical or mechanical/appliance-based solutions. Unless a functional approach like breathing retraining is also taken, a disturbed baseline pattern of breathing may not be addressed at all.

The aim is to normalise the breathing pattern
People are taught to breathe at the correct rate, rhythm and volume and with the correct use of the breathing muscles. The intent is to *retrain* – that

is, *recondition* or *reprogram* – the respiratory centre to operate at the correct level, at rest, when exercising or while sleeping. When it is reset to a more normal set point, improved breathing is maintained day and night.

Breathing is retrainable – habits can be changed

Research has verified that changing breathing habits can reprogram the respiratory centre in the brain. Retraining your breathing is possible because breathing is an automatic body function that can also be voluntarily controlled. Think of your brain as having a manual over-ride and reset button.

Breathing retraining is an essential (not alternative) approach

Breathing ability, efficiency and control is essential to the management of sleep-breathing disorders (and other disorders where dysfunctional breathing is characteristic). Therefore, educating and training people to breathe correctly should be part of a mainstream, not alternative, approach in the management of sleep-breathing disorders.

There are many peer-reviewed studies that show the effectiveness of breathing retraining in normalising dysfunctional breathing patterns.[10.1–10.6] Breathing retraining is also complementary to medical treatment and can be used alongside other treatments. Making nose-breathing more comfortable can help with tolerance of oral splints, and as explained in the previous chapter, CPAP therapy may become more tolerable.

DEFINING BREATHING RETRAINING

Breathing retraining is just one form of 'breath work'. Instruction in breathing is given within many disciplines, including physiotherapy, speech pathology, psychology, singing, yoga, tai chi, qigong, Pilates, and athletic and fitness training. Each has its particular concepts, instructions and exercises, and its own take on why they are important and what they are trying to achieve.

What I refer to throughout this book as *breathing training* or *breathing retraining* may be substantially different in principle and practice from breath work and breathing exercises taught in other disciplines.

Breathing retraining is the specific discipline in which the primary goal is to normalise each aspect of the breathing pattern (rate, rhythm, volume, mechanics, use of the nose), for all situations (awake, asleep, at rest, during eating, speech and exercise). This is a very important definition.

Other disciplines may promote aspects of normal breathing like, for example, slow diaphragm-breathing, but may also encourage large tidal volumes, breathing through the mouth and emptying the lungs. Instruction might include 'take big deep breaths', 'fill your lungs to capacity', 'breathe out as fully as you can', 'breathe out as much carbon dioxide as possible', 'open your mouth, push the air out'.

Training aimed at normalising your baseline breathing pattern is quite different from therapeutic or 'special purpose' breathing exercises that you might do in hospital, in meditation, yoga or Pilates classes, or using various breathing devices. These may have particular aims such as clearing mucous, completely filling or expanding the bases of the lungs, relaxation, 'centring the mind', 'strengthening the core' or strengthening breathing muscles. When the term 'breathing retraining' is used in this book, I am referring only to exercises where the specific goal and design is to achieve physiologically *normal* breathing.

A breathing retraining teacher will want to see that in the minutes, hours, days and nights after a breathing training session, you are breathing closer to a normal pattern. For many people that will mean easier nose-breathing and breathing more regularly, slowly, quietly, efficiently and comfortably – and breaths that take in considerably less air.

WHO TEACHES BREATHING RETRAINING?

As a distinct discipline, breathing retraining is still relatively new and the number of teachers and practitioners is small but growing. They come from various backgrounds; in my case, it was physiotherapy. When I refer in this book to *breathing teachers/educators*, I mean specifically those who teach breathing retraining as defined above (see Chapter 27).

THE BREATHING RETRAINING PROCESS

Assessment, education and training are all components of the breathing retraining process. Assessment identifies poor breathing habits, symptoms and triggers. It looks at breathing mechanics, use of the breathing muscles and breathing rhythm.

Education includes some basic anatomy and physiology to give an understanding of the breathing process and how it impacts the way different body systems function. Posture, diet, behaviours and lifestyle factors that influence breathing are covered, as well as specific breathing retraining instructions and exercises. These include exercises to help reduce nasal stuffiness, irritable cough, shortness of breath and feelings of panic.

The techniques also assist in establishing gentle, rhythmic diaphragm-breathing and in reconditioning the set point of breathing. This helps maintain a healthy breathing pattern and prevent symptoms in the long term. Breathing retraining also provides a foundation for fitness activities.

Improvements in daytime breathing patterns help prevent disordered breathing during sleep. There are various guidelines for sleep, stress, eating, talking, singing and exercising. You can practice while sitting, standing, during movement and during speech. The exercises are not physically demanding and are tailored to the individual. 'Informal practice' is very important – incorporating better breathing into normal daily activities.

THE BUTEYKO METHOD OF BREATHING RETRAINING

The system of breathing retraining developed by medical scientist and physician Professor Konstantin Buteyko is the most succinct, potent, and scientifically sound that I have come across in my extensive research. In the hands of a skilled teacher this method gives a systematic and reliable means of achieving and maintaining healthy breathing and has formed a substantial part of my clinical work.

This particular method of breathing retraining was developed in Russia in the late 1950s. It is based on decades of research and clinical practice by Professor Buteyko. He put together a package of practices that work together to normalise dysfunctional breathing. The Buteyko method was brought to Australia in 1990 and since then has been introduced to many countries.

A typical program involves an initial consultation then a structured program of five to eight 90-minute sessions (60-minute sessions for children). The first five sessions are often done on consecutive days. The instruction may be individual or in small group sessions. The exercises and techniques should be practised on a daily basis, formally and informally, until the breathing pattern is normal and stable, or until people reach the best point they are capable of within the confines of their condition. The exercises can then be tapered down to maintain the improvements.

To achieve their best, people with a mild breathing disorder may need only a week or two of formal practice; moderate cases may need three to eight weeks, and severe cases may need three months to a year.

Medical reappraisal

Clients who undergo breathing retraining are advised to go to their doctor for reappraisal of their condition generally and in particular when significant change is seen in their breathing pattern and symptoms. Clients are advised that changes in prescribed medication and treatments must be undertaken only in consultation with their doctor. A follow-up sleep study is recommended for clients with sleep-breathing disorders (see Chapter 25).

BENEFITS OF BREATHING RETRAINING

Normalising breathing can have physical, mechanical, physiological and biochemical effects. You may benefit generally from enhanced oxygenation and a calming effect on the nervous system. Various body functions may improve, and with that, many symptoms associated with breathing pattern dysfunction can resolve. The processes involved are explained in Chapters 6 and 7.

The benefits listed below typify those reported by my clients, their family members, their doctors and healthcare professionals, 'before and after' scans, tests and sleep study reports.

Commonly reported benefits or changes after undertaking a breathing retraining program include:

- ability to nose-breathe
- less mucous and congestion
- shrinkage of polyps
- improved quality of sleep
- fewer instances or cessation of snoring
- quieter or silent breathing
- fewer breathing stoppages/apnoea
- fewer episodes of gasping and choking
- less waking and sleep disturbance
- fewer overnight toilet trips
- refreshing sleep
- reduced leg twitching/restless legs
- mouth and throat not as dry on waking
- decreased muscle soreness on waking
- greater muscle and general relaxation
- fewer early morning headaches
- more stamina for daytime activities
- easier breathing at rest, during sleep and exercise
- improved exercise capacity
- faster recovery from physical exertion
- less anxiety and tension
- decline in asthma and sinus symptoms
- fewer colds
- improved general health
- improved focus and concentration.

Many people respond in the first session. Stuffy noses usually improve quickly; many sleep better and more quietly right from the first night. My records show that by the fifth session, the majority of snorers and sleep apnoea sufferers have less daytime sleepiness and fatigue and, according to partner feedback, significantly reduced snoring and apnoea episodes. Although it may take weeks or even months to achieve the best breathing pattern possible, clients more often than not experience a dramatic improvement in symptoms within the first five days.

> *Gregory had been snoring for as long as he (and his family) could remember. His wife rated his snoring as being at least eight out of ten in terms of intensity. He had a lot of congestion and more often than not his nose was blocked throughout the day and night. After his first consultation he noticed that his mucous decreased. On the third night of his course he found that he slept eight hours straight without needing the usual overnight toilet visit. He felt totally refreshed and clear-headed in the morning. His wife came home after being away for three weeks and she thought he had died in his sleep! He was the quietest he had been in 40 years.*

The figures for changes in respiration and heart rates in Table 10.1 and for total Symptom Scores in Table 10.2 are taken from my records. They are typical for adults attending my breathing retraining programs, where the first five sessions are done on consecutive days. Some participants used the special Buteyko breathing techniques, others did not.

LONG-TERM RESULTS

How far and fast someone progresses in improving their breathing depends on the extent of breathing disturbance, their underlying health conditions, their level of self-awareness, motivation and commitment, their attention to lifestyle factors that influence breathing and on the skill of their teacher, if they have one (see also Chapter 26).

Once your breathing set point is at a more optimal level, it should stay there, providing there is no return to poor breathing habits, or to lifestyle choices that adversely affect your breathing. In essence, breathing retraining is an educative and self-managed approach. And isn't it great to know that a better functioning body and a healthier life is something you can have control over?

Now let me provide you with tools that thousands of my clients have found effective in improving their breathing, boosting their energy, and in restoring quiet, restful sleep.

TABLE 10.1: RESPIRATION AND HEART RATES

	Day one	Day five
Average resting respiration rate	16	11
Average resting heart rate	78	63
Average respiration rate after two mins moderate-pace walking	19	13
Average heart rate after two mins moderate-pace walking	93	68

TABLE 10.2: SYMPTOM SCORE REDUCTIONS

	Day five	Follow-on session (Approx. day ten)
Average reduction in Symptom Score	60–69%	73–82%

PART TWO
HOW TO CHANGE YOUR BREATHING:
DAY BY DAY, HABIT BY HABIT

*'Everyone thinks of changing the world, but
no one thinks of changing himself.'*

LEO TOLSTOY

CHAPTER 11

Nine healthy breathing habits in five days

Now it's time to develop the good breathing habits you have been reading about and learn how to apply them in your daily life. This program can be implemented in as little as five days, and the aim is to get you to breathe quietly, gently and rhythmically (see Figure 11.1). Figure 11.2 shows the nine healthy breathing habits.

FIGURE 11.1: THE AIM OF THE FIVE-DAY PROGRAM

OUR AIM IS TO CHANGE THIS:

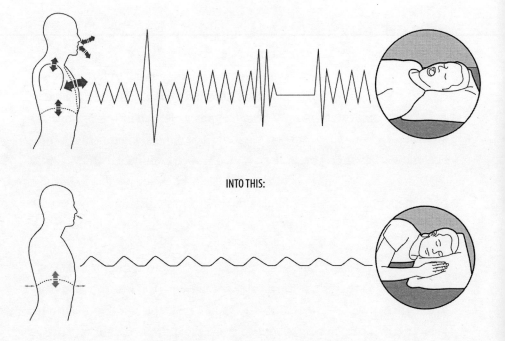

INTO THIS:

FIGURE 11.2: THE NINE HEALTHY BREATHING HABITS

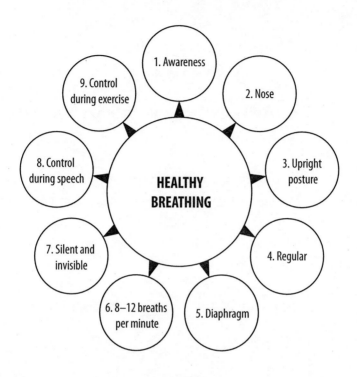

FIVE-DAY PROGRAM TO BETTER BREATHING

These healthy breathing habits can be learnt over a five-day program. And that's not every hour of every day that you have to devote to formal exercises. It can be just five to ten minutes here and there throughout the day.

With familiarity, a lot of the practice can be blended into your normal activities. In fact, that is the best way. Like speaking a different language, becoming a better breather is best done through continual attention and application in everyday situations until it becomes a regular, reflexive habit. Repetition is what develops a habit. In an astonishingly short space of time, a lifetime of destructive breathing habits can be transformed. How good is that?

Most people can make great progress by following the program as per Table 11.1. That is not to say they will have perfect breathing by day five, but they will know the how-to. After that, the healthy breathing habits need to continue to be applied to everyday life, and to be practised daily until the best breathing pattern possible is achieved and becomes second nature. That is days for some, and weeks, months, or even a year for others. Some people require more days at each stage, especially if they have complicating factors, such as anxiety, serious illness, or dysfunctional breathing with significantly disturbed body chemistry. The level of improvement also depends on the amount of time you give to practice, what posture you start out with, your diet and which medications you take. Also, some people learn very well from a book but others may need the attention of a teacher to make a breakthrough.

The order in which the habits are presented is usually the best sequence to work through them. There are suggestions, however, for changing the order if you struggle with any particular habit. The habits from the previous day are continued as you introduce new ones.

TABLE 11.1: THE TYPICAL FIVE-DAY PROGRAM

Day one	Awareness
	Nose-breathing
	Posture
Day two and day three	Regular breathing
	Diaphragm-breathing
Day four	Silent, invisible breathing
	Breathing control during speech
Day five	Breathing well during exercise

Notice that healthy habit six (breathing eight to twelve breaths a minute) is not listed in this program guide. That's because it doesn't have to be practised. It normally develops naturally from implementing the other habits. So that's one less thing to do.

It is recommended that you read through all the information in each section. Even if you see the heading and think 'I'm right with nose-breathing/posture/diaphragm-breathing,' please read through to be absolutely sure. Why? Because unconscious mouth-breathing, especially during activity, is really common; your idea of good posture may not match mine; and many people practise diaphragm-breathing, but it is often woefully incorrect.

People frequently notice an improvement in their sleep and a reduction in snoring from developing the first three habits. By the time you introduce the fourth and fifth habits, the signs of snoring and apnoea may be significantly reduced. It is strongly recommended, however, that you address all nine habits for the sake of long-term and lasting benefits, not only in the quality of your sleep, but also in general health. Breathing correctly will give you a wonderful tool to withstand the stresses of modern living. Think of it as a form of health insurance.

Due to sleep deprivation, adults and children can show signs of forgetfulness and difficulty learning new things. In the early days of breathing retraining, some people find it easier to practise better breathing while standing or walking around to stop them falling asleep!

Remember:

- You may need to check with your doctor before beginning breathing retraining.
- Read each section and implement the changes and the action steps.
- Move on to the next section when the previous habit is 'second nature', or when guided to do so.
- Seek help from a breathing teacher if you struggle to instil the correct habits.
- Stop the implementation of the new breathing habit, at least for the time being, if you experience a negative response. Follow the suggestions given and seek guidance from a doctor and breathing teacher if necessary.
- See your doctor for reassessment of any sleep-breathing condition before discontinuing or changing any prescribed treatments (see Chapter 25).

CHAPTER 12

Healthy habit one: Awareness

The first step in improving your breathing is to be aware of the way you breathe, and how it compares to normal, healthy breathing – nasal, smooth, satisfying, silent, small, slow, low and 'still'. You have to notice your breathing faults before you can work on undoing them. Without this connection, you will struggle to make the changes.

Back in Chapter 4 you went through the self-assessment process – now is a good time to have a quick look again at what you wrote down in Table 4.1. By now you are likely more aware of your breathing and perhaps have already made some changes – possibly doing less mouth-breathing. However, when you put this book down and go about your business, without some level of mindfulness, you are likely to revert to bad habits. Many people think they are completely nose-breathing during the daytime until they start paying close attention – then they discover they breathe through their mouth when walking, showering, concentrating, pegging out the washing, getting up from a chair and getting in and out of the car.

OBSERVATION CHECKLIST

Tune in to the rate, rhythm, sound, route (mouth or nose) and location of your breathing. An 'all-the-time' general awareness is best, but to help you achieve this, I suggest you schedule yourself a formal spot-check once every (waking) hour for a few days.

Watch out for the particular breathing 'faults' in the left-hand column of the Observations Checklist (Table 12.1, page 95) and place an X in each box where you notice them occurring in a certain situation. I suggest you carry this book or a photocopy of that page with you for the next few days – until you feel it is second nature to be aware of your breathing.

GETTING FEEDBACK

This can be very useful. So many people have no idea how often they breathe through their mouth, clear their throat, sigh, yawn, sniff or cough. These unconscious habits can, however, be quite obvious, even annoying, to others.

> William only became aware of his habitual cough when he overheard a work colleague identifying him to a new staff member as 'the guy in the cubicle over there who is always coughing'.

Engage the help of family and friends by explaining that you want to be made aware so you can eliminate these habits. (They will probably be thrilled to help.) Give them permission to tell you when your mouth is open or your breathing is fast or noisy, until you're thoroughly aware of these habits. Ask your partner to observe your breathing during sleep. Even if you don't snore, your breathing may be audible, and you may be blowing a gale over your partner.

ACTION STEPS FOR BREATHING AWARENESS
- Generally observe your breathing throughout the day.
- Spot-check your breathing once an hour, using the checklist, for a few days.
- Ask your family or friends to comment on your breathing.

When to move on

You can move on straightaway to healthy habit two: nose-breathing.

TABLE 12.1: OBSERVATIONS CHECKLIST

How am I breathing?	Sitting	Moving about	Under stress	Getting in / out of a car	Lying down	On waking	Showering
Mouth							
Audible							
Fast							
Irregular							
Upper chest							
Breath holding							
Sighing							
Yawning							
Large, full breaths							
Coughing							
Sneezing							
Throat clearing							
Puffing/ Panting							
Gasping when talking							

CHAPTER 13

Healthy habit two: Nose-breathing

The second task is to work towards becoming a full-time nose-breather –
day and night and with exercise.

STRATEGIES FOR DAYTIME NOSE-BREATHING

For many people mouth-breathing is simply a habit or else born of a lack of
awareness. By paying attention to the way you are breathing, you may find
that you can make easy progress. Just consciously try to breathe through
your nose whenever you catch yourself mouth-breathing. Even if nasal
congestion has been a problem, it generally lessens as you reduce your
tendency to over-breathe – through awareness and simply by giving nose-
breathing a go. It usually doesn't take long before you feel a difference.

> *Don was sitting in the back row at one of my information seminars. Towards the end of the
> one-hour session, a lady asked if it was any use her attending breathing retraining sessions
> when she found it impossible to breathe through her nose. Before I could answer, Don leapt
> up from his chair and said, 'Yes! I came in with a totally blocked nose – in fact, I have not
> breathed through my nose for at least 30 years – but I have been breathing through it easily
> for the last fifteen minutes.'*

Here are instructions to help you become a consistent nose-breather.

Instructions

Practice Sets A and B are for those who mouth-breathe but whose noses
are *not* blocked. Set C is for those who have a blocked or congested nose.

PRACTICE SET A: BASIC NOSE-BREATHING INSTRUCTIONS

For those who find nose-breathing comfortable but are just forgetful, aim to progressively increase the total amount of time you nose-breathe each day until you are a 100 per cent nose-breather. How? Simply by being mindful of nose-breathing whenever you can, continuing the awareness you developed in the previous chapter. Keep trying your nose out!

However, don't persist with nose-breathing if you find it distressing. If you are a chronic mouth-breather, you may need to take the transition to nose-breathing very slowly the first few days.

You can be so used to the large amount of air you get via the mouth that you need to recondition yourself to a smaller tidal volume. In this situation a goal of, say, a 5 per cent increase in the total amount of time spent nose-breathing may be enough for the first few days. Most people can cope with that. It usually doesn't take long to begin to adapt.

A very gradual transition like this also may be necessary if you have a head cold or allergic rhinitis or suffer with anxiety or panic disorder. (See page 103 – A message for anxious people.)

- Favour nose-breathing whenever possible so long as it's comfortable.
- Aim to increase your total daytime nose-breathing progressively each day until it's 100 per cent.
- If you almost never nose-breathe and/or your nose feels congested, try to increase your total nose-breathing time by just 5 per cent a day.
- If you feel breathless, panicky or dizzy, leave off the nose-breathing practice for now. You may be able to do it more comfortably next time you sit down to read, or try Set C.
- When/if you have to mouth-breathe make it as gentle as you can.
- Read the sections on nose-breathing during transfers, movement and sleep.
- If after two days you have made no progress, try Practice Set B or C.

PRACTICE SET B: NOSE-BREATHING IS UNCOMFORTABLE BUT YOUR NOSE IS NOT BLOCKED

If you don't feel you are making substantial progess with nose-breathing try the following:

1. Determine how long you can maintain nose-breathing before needing to take a breath (not a gasp) through your mouth. Let's say, for example, fifteen seconds.
2. Go back to (very gentle) mouth-breathing for 30 seconds.
3. Nose-breathe again and try to add an extra five to ten seconds before reverting to gentle mouth-breathing again for 30 seconds.
4. Repeat three more times or until the five minutes is up.

Try to increase the time you nose-breathe in each cycle: from fifteen seconds to twenty seconds, 30 seconds, 35 seconds, 45 seconds. After five minutes total, take a break for an hour and then start the routine again. When you can comfortably breathe for 60 seconds continuously through your nose, try cutting down (or out), the 30-second mouth-breathing breaks until you can comfortably and continuously nose-breathe for the whole five minutes. Hopefully you can then keep up nose-breathing throughout your next activity.

Aim to do this conscious practice once every waking hour until you are converted to continuous nose-breathing while sitting down. You can practise while watching TV, standing in a queue, sitting in a waiting room or on the bus. If at any time you feel distress or panic, take a break and try again later.

PRACTICE SET C: YOUR NOSE FEELS BLOCKED

If you feel as if no air goes in when you try to nose-breathe, try a *short breath hold* (SBH). This is a technique where after a normal (not forced) exhalation, you pause your breath for one to three seconds, then breathe slowly and gently for three or four breaths. Then you repeat the pattern. The slight increase in carbon dioxide that occurs seems to soothe swollen nasal membrane tissue.

The pause should not be so long as to alter the breathing pattern after the pause. That is, the breaths afterwards must be gentle, or at least not bigger or deeper than before (see Figure 13.1). If you hold too long and stimulate increased breathing, you lose the beneficial effect of the slight rise in carbon dioxide.

1. After a natural out-breath, pause your breath for one to three seconds.
2. Start breathing – as *gently* as you can – through your nose if it's clear or your mouth if it's not.
3. Repeat the pause after every third or fourth out-breath.
4. Follow this routine for three to five minutes.

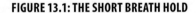

FIGURE 13.1: THE SHORT BREATH HOLD

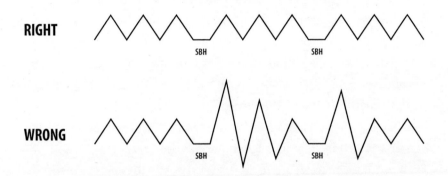

When first nose-breathing, you may feel like barely any air is getting through, but hopefully your nose will gradually clear, with the nose-breaths delivering an increasingly satisfying feeling. The gentler the nose- and mouth-breaths, the faster this effect should be felt. Repeat Set C once per waking hour if you can, gradually increasing the time spent on the routine to ten minutes. Once you find that your nose is no longer block-ing up between practice times, you can try Set B.

If at any stage, during either Set B or Set C, you feel distress, panic, breathlessness or light-headedness, or you find yourself taking bigger mouth-breaths, stop the practice, recover and breathe comfortably – however you must. Take a break and come back later or resume practice at a level of nose-breathing time or short breath hold time that you were comfortable with, and stay there until you feel ready to progress. It is very important that the nose-breathing periods are *not* followed by deep breaths through your mouth. If they are, you have pushed yourself too far. Don't force the inhales or the exhales.

Also try nose-breathing during movement – Set D. By moving about slowly enough, you may even find it is easier than nose-breathing while sitting.

Still mouth-breathing? At least make it gentle

When you do have to mouth-breathe, try to do it more gently, taking in less air than you used to. This will also help improve your breathing – not as quickly as completely switching to nose-breathing, but you will still be acclimatising to less air and becoming a more efficient breather. You may find you can be quite satisfied without sucking in as much air as you used to.

There are some additional strategies if needed on page 106.

NOSE-BREATHING DURING MOVEMENT

Establishing nose-breathing during light activity is very important. When you first switch from mouth-breathing to nose-breathing, this will most likely require you to walk and do day-to-day activities more slowly. Slow down to a pace at which you can *comfortably* nose-breathe; don't push yourself into discomfort.

You may feel like you have to move at a snail's pace at first to achieve this, but it can make an incredible difference to your overall progress with improving your breathing. Allow yourself more time to get places – across the room, out to the garage, up the stairs, to your seat at the football (and more time to wash yourself in the shower). The payoff is that you should be less breathless when you get there, and need less or no recovery time. Most people have their speed back within a few days.

If you are reasonably active, you will find that before long, walking up stairs and hills, housework, gardening and lawn mowing become easier and you should have less or no huffing and puffing. Not only that, but breathing in a more controlled way as you go about your day should translate into more stable breathing during sleep.

On the other hand, if you don't attend to this, you can severely hamper your progress. Remember, you do need more air when you are moving, so it is natural to take fuller or deeper breaths – but these should still be through your nose. Let it happen naturally, though – neither restrict the amount of air you take in through your nose nor exaggerate it by deliberately trying to take in more air. As always, comfortable is the operative word.

The golden rule of nose-breathing: *Go only as fast as your nose will comfortably allow.*

Instructions

Try this routine, taking into account your usual exercise capacity.

PRACTICE SET D: NOSE-BREATHING DURING MOVEMENT

1. Start with a three-minute leisurely walk on flat ground.
2. Pace yourself when walking so that you can breathe comfortably in and out of your nose. (*Comfortably* – not torturously.)
3. If you feel breathless, or that you must open your mouth, slow down, walk even more slowly, or stop and rest until nose-breathing is comfortable again. Then start walking again at a slower pace.
4. Once you have found the pace that you can comfortably nose-breathe at, try to nose-breathe during all your walking and usual physical activities: climbing stairs, bending, lifting, and getting in and out of the car.
5. Increase your walking speed, distance and the incline as your breathing improves.

If your exercise capacity is quite low, adjust your movement goal accordingly. Don't give up if you are unable to do this on your own. Stay with it as much as possible and get extra help, if you can, from a breathing teacher. I accompany elderly clients (including some using portable oxygen cylinders) to their cars after their appointments, and they're often amazed by how much easier the walk is when they are consciously nose-breathing. We may take a little longer than usual to get to the car, but once there, the clients do not need to recover from breathlessness.

For those with average exercise capacity

When nose-breathing during walking is second nature, introduce it into other forms of exercise, such as cycling or using the treadmill or rowing machine at the gym. Again, choose a pace at which you can maintain comfortable nose-breathing.

You may need to push your bike up hills for the first few days. This can be frustrating, but it is very important in the training process. In the long run, your breathing becomes more efficient and you will soon get back to your old speed. Because you are oxygenating better, you may well end up going faster than before.

> Amanda, twelve, was referred for breathing retraining by her dentist. Her chronic mouth-breathing had led to a narrow upper palate and crowded teeth. She snored like a trooper, but had no nasal blockage. I timed how long she could breathe through her nose: after just two seconds, her mouth flew open and she exclaimed that she felt like she was suffocating. Through breathing retraining, Amanda quickly adjusted to needing less air. By day three, she was comfortably nose-breathing all day and night. On day five she easily jogged 400m and then sprinted 200m with her mouth closed.

How to breathe well during exercise, sport and strenuous physical activity will be covered more fully in Chapter 20.

NOSE-BREATHING DURING TRANSFERS

People commonly revert to mouth-breathing when changing position or situation – during 'transfers' – like getting up from a chair, going from a warm house into cold air, getting in and out of the shower or car, or bending down to put their socks on. Doing a short breath hold of one to three seconds while you transfer can be extremely useful in preventing mouth-breathing and breathlessness.

STRATEGIES FOR NOSE-BREATHING DURING SLEEP

Anything that increases your breathing rate in the day or evening may affect the tendency to mouth-breathe at night and exacerbate sleep-disordered breathing. Here are some suggestions to prevent over-breathing and to facilitate nose-breathing during sleep.

Nose-breathe all day

The more you nose-breathe during the day, the better you'll adapt to a smaller tidal volume and the more likely you'll be to continue nose-breathing while asleep. You'll also reduce the likelihood of nasal congestion.

Practise nose-breathing before bed

Practise nose-breathing Set B or C for two five-minute periods (with a one-minute rest in between) during the half-hour before bed.

Sleep on your side

The position of heaviest breathing during sleep is flat on your back with your mouth open, and arms up over your head – the 'open mouth, open chest' position. Snorers are almost invariably louder on their backs (*supine*).

When you are asleep, your muscles are more relaxed, and when you're on your back, your lower jaw is more likely to drop open. Most

---

A MESSAGE FOR ANXIOUS PEOPLE – DON'T PANIC!

Long-term mouth-breathers and people who experience claustrophobia, anxiety or panic attacks may have feelings of panic when they initially attempt nose-breathing. For some, just sitting with their mouth closed for a couple of seconds can make them feel panicky. This is likely because they are conditioned to breathing a large volume of air and having a correspondingly low carbon dioxide level. The sudden increase in carbon dioxide when they breathe less (shut their mouth) can cause a reaction. It is important then to make changes very gradually to allow the body time to adjust.

I have found the best way to begin is with informal practice as in Set A – where you set a goal to spend just 5 per cent more time each day breathing through your nose. This is a very gentle yet profound way of achieving continuous nose-breathing. In my experience, most people with anxiety states are comfortable with daytime nose-breathing within a week by starting off like this. Don't stress; slow and steady wins the race.

For some anxious clients, a change first in posture (Chapter 14) or diet (Chapter 22) is helpful. If none of these suggestions help, consult your doctor, who may be able to find another cause for an elevated drive to breathe or help you to access treatment for unresolved psychological issues that may underlie your breathing-pattern disturbance.

sleep studies show more snoring, hypopnoea and apnoea episodes occur during supine sleeping. Many people find their breathing is most gentle when lying on the left side. Special pillows can be purchased that prevent you sleeping on your back, or else you can wedge pillows behind you. One client with a really intransigent back-sleeping habit trained himself to stay on his side by wearing a backpack stuffed with a football!

Sleep with your upper body elevated

The flatter you lie, generally the deeper (larger) you breathe, the more effort it takes, and the more likely you are to breathe through your mouth.

Elevating the head end of the bed about 10 cm (or even more) in the early stages of breathing retraining (or when you have a cold), can make nose-breathing easier (see Figure 13.2). This can be done by placing a folded blanket between the mattress and bed base, packing pillows in a wedge shape or using specially designed foam wedges to elevate your upper body. Be careful when using extra pillows not to bend your neck in such a way as to contribute to snoring or neck pain. A flat mattress with just one pillow is usually quite sufficient for people who breathe correctly.

Please note: Although side-sleeping is the preferred position for better breathing, there are spinal, musculoskeletal and other medical conditions that make this sleeping position inadvisable. Please consult your doctor or health-care provider if you are unsure.

FIGURE 13.2: ELEVATED SIDE-SLEEPING

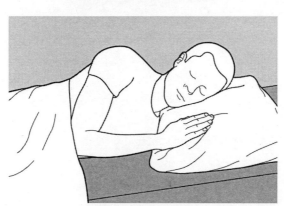

Try a chin strap

If you are comfortable with nose-breathing, but your mouth tends to drop open during sleep, a *chin strap* may help. Chin straps are made from cloth, with a pouch-like support under the chin and an adjustable head strap. They are designed to help keep your mouth closed while you sleep. Chin straps are available online, from some pharmacies, or through the same companies that make CPAP equipment.

> Chin straps, special pillows and bed elevation should be looked on as interim aids to assist with developing a nose-breathing pattern at night. They are not meant to be a substitute for conscious efforts to increase mindfulness of nose-breathing and normalise your breathing pattern.

Avoid smoking and second-hand smoke

Smoke inhalation can contribute to nasal and lung congestion. Nicotine also relaxes muscles and may contribute to poor muscle tone during sleep.

Other things to avoid in the evening

The following can cause you to 'breathe up':

- caffeinated drinks and chocolate.
- exercising within three hours of bedtime: exercise increases your body temperature and breathing rate and when taken too close to bedtime may increase a tendency to insomnia or snoring.
- eating within two to three hours of bedtime: digestion promotes increased metabolic activity and increased breathing rate.
- large meals with a lot of animal protein and/or high-starch/high-sugar content (see Chapter 22 for more detail).
- alcohol before bed: your breathing rate may increase as alcohol is metabolised. This, combined with alcohol's relaxing effect on the throat dilator muscles, increases the likelihood of snoring and apnoea. Avoiding alcohol for the first few days of this program can help you make headway in bringing your breathing under control.
- over-heating: make sure your bedroom is not overly warm and that you are not wearing too much clothing or using more blankets than necessary.

- over-sleeping: breathing tends to get heavier towards morning. Headache, nasal congestion and fatigue can be the unwelcome result of a sleep-in. What a way to start the day! It is best to sleep only when you are tired, and to get up as soon as you wake in the morning. For most adults seven to eight hours of quality sleep per night is enough. As your breathing improves, you may find you wake earlier. If you go back to sleep again you are more likely to wake later with signs of over-breathing.

> Eve noticed that she was waking up at 5.30 a.m. feeling refreshed and with a clear nose, but when she decided to get some extra sleep, she would wake again around 7 a.m. feeling tired and blocked up.

EXTRA STRATEGIES FOR UNBLOCKING 'RESISTANT' NOSES
Diet change

Persistent nasal congestion often responds to a change in diet, particularly a reduction in milk (for some) and high-starch/high-sugar foods (such as chocolate, desserts, pastries, cakes, cereal, bread, pasta and rice). The connection between breathing and diet is covered in Chapter 22.

Saline nasal sprays

The mucous membranes lining the nose need to be kept moist to effectively clear the inhaled air of dust, germs and pollens. This protective role is compromised when the air is too dry, like in an aircraft, or when you are dehydrated through over-breathing. If you suffer from long-term nasal congestion, you may benefit from using a saline (salt and water) nasal spray. These are available from pharmacies.

Salt solutions are valued for their antiseptic, anti-inflammatory and anti-allergen properties. Unlike some of the medicated decongestant sprays, saline nasal sprays do not cause rebound congestion. The effect is not dissimilar to the great nose-clearing effect experienced when you swim in the ocean. Nasal congestion usually responds quickly to breathing retraining and nasal sprays are not usually needed on an ongoing basis.

Nasal medications

There are various prescription and over-the-counter medications for nasal problems – in spray, tablet or inhaler forms. There are the 'reliever' or decongestant types that shrink the nasal linings, and 'preventer' types that are anti-allergen or anti-inflammatory. Speak to your doctor or pharmacist about the appropriate type for you and correct usage. Overuse of the medicated decongestants can cause rebound congestion.

NEED MORE HELP?

The exercises and suggestions in this book are not a guaranteed solution for all nasal passage problems. Seeing a breathing teacher may help you make a breakthrough if you have a really chronic problem that is over-breathing related. However, some nasal problems do require surgery or medications.

Consult your doctor if you suspect you have a nasal or sinus infection. Also be aware that successful long-term treatment of sinusitis may need to incorporate treatment of any infections situated around teeth and their roots.

TIMEFRAME

The time it should take to achieve 100 per cent nose-breathing will vary according to many factors, including the nature, severity and duration of the problem, your level of awareness, your commitment to practising, and which medical treatments you have had or currently use. Even your sleeping position, posture and diet are factors. In other words, results will differ for each individual.

In my experience, most people can break a mouth-breathing habit within two to five days, providing any nasal obstruction is not primarily structural, and it rarely is. Your progress can be even faster when undergoing breathing retraining sessions with a teacher, as they can provide more intensive or individually tailored training in a supervised setting.

It is not uncommon for me to see people who are on the waiting list to see an ear, nose and throat specialist breathing freely through their nose halfway through their first breathing session! (They do, however, need more time than that to completely break the habit.) Many clients have reported that polyps and adenoids have reduced in size following breathing retraining, and this has been verified by scans and physical examinations.

SORE NOSES AND NASAL SNORING

Breathing through your nose does not necessarily mean that your breathing is perfect. Your tidal volume and airflow rate can still be too high. While it is a big step in the right direction for a mouth-breather, nasal over-breathing can still result in mucous and irritation in the nasal passages. You may be accused of noisy breathing during the day and nasal snoring at night. As you develop the rest of the healthy habits, your breathing slows, softens and quietens. (Then your partner may at first be 'spooked' by the eerie silence.)

Some people experience discomfort in the nose when they first convert to nose-breathing. The nasal lining has not been exposed to continuous airflow like this for a long time, maybe decades, maybe never, and can be hypersensitive at first. This too will pass.

ACTION STEPS FOR NOSE-BREATHING (DAYTIME)

- Awareness – spot-check yourself for mouth-breathing.
- Try to breathe only through your nose.
- Aim to increase the percentage of time you nose-breathe each day.
- Let your ability to comfortably nose-breathe dictate the pace of walking and activities.
- Go slow now to be faster later.
- If you have to mouth-breathe, do so as gently as you can.

- Close your mouth and pause breathing for one to three seconds during transfers.
- Refer to the dietary guidelines on page 105 and in Chapter 22.
- Practise Set B or C once every waking hour until continuous nose-breathing is easy.

ACTION STEPS FOR NOSE-BREATHING (NIGHT-TIME)

- Nose-breathe during the day.
- Sleep with your upper body slightly elevated.
- Avoid sleeping on your back.
- Sleep with your mouth closed.
- Consider wearing a chin strap.
- Avoid exercising within three hours of bedtime.
- Allow two to three hours after eating before bed.
- Avoid large meals of an evening.
- Avoid alcohol at night.
- Avoid high-starch/high-sugar meals.
- Avoid over-heating and over-sleeping.
- Practise Set B or C for two five-minute periods before bed.
- Consider a saline nasal spray in the initial stages.

When to move on

You can move on straightaway to healthy habit three: upright posture, as it will help you move closer to 100 per cent nose-breathing. Just keep up the strategies and practice as above until nose-breathing at rest, while sleeping and during activity become second nature.

If nose-breathing remains uncomfortable, as well as moving on to the next chapter, the suggestions in Chapter 22 may be helpful.

Even if you must continue to mouth-breathe because your health condition will not allow comfortable nose-breathing, there are still many benefits to be had by making improvements in the other breathing habits, as they may enhance your breathing mechanics and efficiency. Even mouth-breathing gently and in more controlled manner than you used to is a terrific step forward.

CHAPTER 14

Healthy habit three: Upright posture

I hope I haven't caught you here glued to this book, sitting with your shoulders slouched, abdomen folded over, head down, chin forward – and breathing using your upper chest!

The diaphragm is the main muscle for breathing and its action is compromised with a slumped posture. When you are 'folded over', you are compressing the lower chest and the abdomen. Your breathing rate and level of tension increase, and so does the likelihood of upper-chest breathing, mouth-breathing and over-breathing. Once the chest muscles get over-involved, breathing volume goes up by 50–80 per cent.

On the other hand, good posture optimises your breathing mechanics. When combined with nose-breathing, it automatically facilitates diaphragmatic breathing. That's why, despite how important diaphragm-breathing is, it's not at the top of the list in terms of learning to breathe correctly.

Unfortunately, there are several myths about good posture – so please don't skip this section thinking you already know all about it! First, good posture is not about straightness and stiffness. Second, it is not about effort.

STRATEGIES FOR GOOD POSTURE
The coathanger posture – the relaxed, lengthened upright posture
I have found the concept of the coathanger posture to be a simple and effective way to develop better posture and to 'unfold' and 'open up' the typical slumped posture. I also use the notions of letting go and allowing – relaxing and letting the correct positions and movements to simply happen. These concepts are more about undoing than consciously doing

one, which often creates tension and effort. Some of these ideas are also part of the Alexander technique, an educational modality that assists in achieving good posture and free body movement.

> **THE SLUMP TEST**
>
> After a minute sitting relaxed with an upright posture, feel where your breathing movement is. Then collapse your posture and deliberately sit slumped over. Now notice the movement again. (Breathing usually goes to the upper chest.) Now please sit upright and stay there!

Instructions for sitting

Choose a firm chair of a height that allows your thighs to be parallel to the ground (and slightly apart), your knees bent at a right angle and your feet flat on the floor. Your hands rest in your lap. Now imagine having a coathanger inside you – the hook part inside your head and the shoulder framework within your shoulder area. Imagine that your coathanger is hung on a railing that's at the perfect height for you.

Imagine your body is supported by, and draping from, the internal coathanger, so that you can just relax and soften your muscles, let go, and allow yourself to lengthen in two directions: up through the crown of your head; down through your sit bones (the bony knobs in your buttocks) into the chair. Think of your neck as part of your torso. When you get the relaxation and 'letting go' right, you may feel your pelvis drop slightly away from your chest. The net effect you are aiming for is *relaxed, lengthened sitting* (see Figure 14.1).

It is very important to let go of tension in your shoulders and to have a soft, relaxed stomach. Your face muscles and jaw also need to be relaxed. Say to yourself, 'Long face, soft jaw'. Have your lips touching but your teeth apart.

The idea of the coathanger posture is that it allows the body to relax while at the same time not collapsing and losing any height. This feels very different to the tension created by the usual 'sit up straight' command. How does it feel? Most people feel relaxed; their breathing movement reduces, and breaths are slow and quiet, dropping automatically from the upper chest to the lower rib cage/diaphragm area.

This posture also helps you settle your breathing quickly when distressed. I have put these instructions into the list below. It may help to record yourself slowly reading it through and then play it back as you sit in the coathanger posture. (See also Learning resources – Audio aids to learning, page 231.)

FIGURE 14.1: SITTING IN THE COATHANGER POSTURE

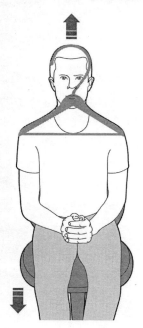

PRACTICE SET: RELAXED, LENGTHENED SITTING

How to take up the coathanger posture:

1. Feet flat on the floor; thighs parallel to the ground.
2. Hands relaxed in your lap.
3. Imagine your coathanger in position.
4. Let go of the long muscles down either side of the spine.
5. Allow your neck to soften and lengthen.
6. Allow your body to soften and lengthen – up through your head, down through your sit bones.
7. Relax your shoulders; allow them to soften, widen and drop.
8. Soften your stomach muscles.
9. Relax your jaw; have your lips together, your teeth apart.
10. Keep your face long, and your jaw soft.

11. Sit in this position and breathe as gently as you can, through your nose, for three to five minutes.

12. If you find this comfortable, then try to extend the time to five to ten minutes.

PRACTICE TIMES

Until good posture is second nature, aim to check your posture every 'seated' hour, on the hour, and do the three to five minutes of formal practice three to four times a day. You can combine this with your nose-breathing practice. The best times to practice are before getting dressed in the morning, before you go to bed, and whenever you have spare time in your day – such as on the train, before a meeting starts, while in a waiting room or while on hold on the phone.

Instructions for standing and walking

Keeping your diaphragm area relaxed and your spine lengthened during all activities – from daily chores to walking to running a marathon – facilitates healthy breathing. The coathanger posture – lengthening upwards through your head and downwards through your tailbone and your feet – can be used equally well with all these activities.

You should progressively work towards keeping this posture all the time. When you first get out of bed in the morning, imagine putting your coathanger in, looping it over that imaginary railing and allowing your body to drape softly, comfortably and at full length from it. Throughout the day give yourself cues, by asking, 'Am I on my coathanger?' Don't forget to check your posture when in the car, especially if you drive a lot. An adjustment to the seat may be needed to reinforce a better posture.

Undoing the damage

People who have had poor posture for years may have compensated for it and have weak or tight muscles and stiff joints. When you first begin to improve your posture while sitting, it can be tiring and feel unnatural.

You may benefit by using pillows to help prop and support you in sitting. While some of us may be able to achieve good posture through awareness and attention, it is desirable for those with conditions like scoliosis to have professional help to achieve the best posture they are capable of. If you need assistance, I highly recommend the Alexander technique. Massage, muscle-release therapies and heat packs may also assist the release of tight tissues.

The benefits

The benefits from improving your posture can be extraordinary and far-reaching. I have seen the correction of poor posture reduce or eliminate many symptoms of chronic over-breathing within 24 hours.

These improvements may be felt across all systems and can include increased capacity to exercise, improved sleep and digestion, and a sense of relaxation and calm. On the other hand, if you continue to maintain a slumped or folded-over posture, your ability to achieve normal breathing is severely hampered.

ACTION STEPS FOR UPRIGHT POSTURE

- Sit, stand and walk with the relaxed, lengthened 'coathanger' posture.
- Check your posture and breathing once every hour.
- Practise relaxed lengthened sitting for three to five minutes, three to four times a day until good posture is automatic.

YOUR KEYWORDS

- Awareness
- Coathanger
- Nose
- Soften
- Let go
- Allow

When to move on

Move on to healthy habit four: regular breathing, when you have had at least one day practising nose-breathing and the relaxed upright posture.

CHAPTER 15

Healthy habit four: Regular breathing

Irregular breathing is common in people with snoring and sleep apnoea. During the day you see the breathing rhythm interrupted by episodes of fast or heavy breathing, sniffing, throat clearing, coughing, sighing, yawning and breath holding (day apnoea). Coughing and throat clearing can evolve into well-practised habits.

Uneven, irregular breathing in the day destabilises your breathing control and in effect can be seen as setting you up for erratic breathing during sleep – varying breath sizes, heavy breathing, snores of varying intensity, speeding up, slowing down, stopping, starting, snorting. Sharp intakes of air while your throat muscles are relaxed can create sufficient suction pressure to draw the walls of the throat in and obstruct airflow. Large, forceful exhales can drop carbon dioxide too far and trigger hypopnoea or apnoea.

Breathing retraining by day aims to bring back control, smoothness and regularity to your breathing, reprogramming your breathing regulator for smoother, gentler, quieter breathing at night.

STRATEGIES FOR SMOOTH, REGULAR BREATHING
Reducing dry, tickly coughing, throat clearing, yawning, sighing
SHORT BREATH HOLD (SBH)

Short breath holds were first introduced in Chapter 13. They can be a valuable tool for inhibiting large and forceful breaths such as dry, tickly coughing, throat clearing, yawning and sighing.

They can also be used for compensation if prevention fails. Short breath holds make up for some of the carbon dioxide lost through these excessively big breaths. The pause in breathing should not be so long as to alter the breathing pattern after the pause. The resultant rise in carbon dioxide is so slight that there is no stimulation of increased breath size.

These short pauses are followed by an attempt to coax your breathing back into a smooth wave pattern to try to prevent further yawning, sighing, coughing and throat clearing.

PROCEDURE FOR PREVENTION – STOP THE LEAK (OF CARBON DIOXIDE)

When you feel you are about to cough, yawn, sigh or clear your throat, try to inhibit it by:

- closing your mouth.
- pausing your breath for one to three seconds (or swallowing once).
- breathing in and out through your nose, as slowly, gently and smoothly as you can, controlling the rhythm and breath size.
- relaxing your breathing and stomach muscles.

Repeat the process if the urge comes again.

PROCEDURE FOR COMPENSATION – REPAIR THE DAMAGE

Use the short breath hold routine straight after a cough, yawn or sigh if you were unable to inhibit it (see Figure 15.1). This way you compensate for the loss of carbon dioxide – and 'repair the damage' – by building it up again. Also, if you cannot block a cough, put your hand over your mouth to prevent yourself from taking a big breath through it.

Remember: do not pause your breath for a length of time that causes the next breath to be excessively large, or means that you gasp or cough as a result. Breathing retraining is about promoting controlled, silent, gentle breaths. It is about avoiding any negative impact on your breathing.

If you have had a chronic irritable cough, this exercise may need to be used quite frequently to overcome the urge to cough. However, as your breathing improves generally and the airway becomes less irritated, the cough should settle.

FIGURE 15.1: SHORT BREATH HOLDS FOR PREVENTION AND COMPENSATION

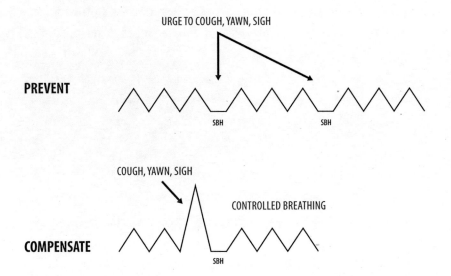

SWALLOW, SIP WATER

A swallow, in place of the short breath hold, or during it, can help you resist a sigh, yawn or cough. Sipping warm water may also help inhibit coughing fits.

Moist, productive coughs

Do not use cough suppression when you need to clear mucous from your airways. However, do try to cough in a more controlled manner. This is particularly important for those with asthma. When mucous needs to be shifted, try to remove it with the minimum amount of coughing that it takes to do so and follow a bout of coughing with nose-breathing – as gentle as possible – and some short breath holds.

When you have to cough, put your hand over your mouth to prevent gulping in so much air, or even try to inhale through your nose, and cough with your mouth closed. This will lessen the irritation on your throat.

If your cough doesn't improve with these suggestions, please consult your doctor. (Even though medications may also help, breathing retraining offers hope for long-term improvement by removing a primary cause of irritation to the trachea and lungs – mouth-breathing/over-breathing.)

> Madeline, a museum guide, used to cough constantly throughout her tours. All the talking she had to do made it worse. Her cough stopped as soon as she started the breathing course. She no longer got exhausted from talking all day, did not have to clear mucous from her throat and did not get dehydrated like she used to.

Sneezing and nose blowing

Because sneezing is involuntary and explosive, it is harder to control than yawning and sighing. It is also not advisable to inhibit a sneeze after the urge and pressure has built up. (Sneezes can be over 100 km/hour.)

Instead, pause your breath for one to three seconds immediately *after* the first sneeze to try to inhibit a series of sneezes. If mucous has accumulated, try to get by with just wiping the end of your nose or with a gentle, small-volume nose blow. Everything connected with breathing should be gentle, including nose blowing. Big honking nose blows will stimulate further mucous production.

PROCEDURE FOR SNEEZING AND NOSE BLOWING
1. Pause your breath for one to three seconds immediately after the first sneeze.
2. Breathe in and out through your nose, as slowly, gently and smoothly as you can, controlling the rhythm and breath size.
3. Try to get by with just wiping your nose or only gentle, small-volume nose blowing.
4. Avoid honking nose blows.

INCREASED YAWNING – THE BATTLE OF THE BREATHING CENTRE

Some people notice an increase in their desire to yawn when they first change their breathing. If you've had chronically low carbon dioxide, which you were maintaining through intermittent sighing, yawning or mouth-breathing, it will take some time for your body to acclimatise.

Your body may at first try to get you over-breathing again and dumping out carbon dioxide in the form of more yawning. It may take a couple of days for the increased desire to yawn to go away. In the meantime, be aware, and do your best to suppress them using a short breath hold or 'swallowing' them.

ACTION STEPS FOR REGULAR BREATHING

- Try to breathe gently and smoothly through your nose at all times.
- Allow no jerkiness or irregularities to disturb the steady flow of your breathing.

COUGHING AND YAWNING

Coughing, because it is so forceful, can be quite abusive to your airway, with each cough further dehydrating and irritating the airway and in turn provoking the next cough. For those with asthma, coughing may provoke bronchospasm. Coughing can also raise your blood pressure and be a strain on your heart. It can be exhausting and difficult to stop.

There are several potential causes of coughing and it is important to have the cause identified and appropriately treated. Moist or 'productive' coughs may or may not be caused by infection. An irritable, dry, tickly, 'unproductive' cough can occur without a medically known cause, but it is certainly exacerbated by mouth-breathing.

Breathing retraining aims to reduce dry, tickly coughing and thereby protect your airways from irritation and excessive physical forces.

No one fully understands why we yawn. Whatever the reason, an odd yawn of an evening, when we are bored or as a copycat behaviour is quite natural and may serve us well. However, repetitive yawning is a marker of dysfunctional breathing and can provoke and perpetuate symptoms.

- Use the short breath hold routine and/or a swallow to prevent or compensate for a yawn, sigh, dry cough, sneeze, or erratic/forceful breaths.
- Try to control your breathing rhythm and breath size afterwards.
- If you must blow your nose, do so very gently.
- If you must cough, do so gently and try to keep your mouth closed, or put your hand over your mouth.
- If you need to breathe through your mouth, make it as smooth and gentle as you possibly can.
- Be diligent while your breathing centre adapts.

When to move on

Making your breathing regular will come from being attentive on a day-to-day level. As long as you are comfortable with nose-breathing and a more upright posture you can move on straightaway to healthy habit five: diaphragm-breathing.

However, if you are prone to anxiety, panic and hyperventilation attacks, changes in your breathing often need to be made at a slower pace than others. Spend one or two extra days on getting your posture and nose-breathing habits right, if you feel you need to.

CHAPTER 16

Healthy habit five: Diaphragm-breathing

Diaphragm-breathing is the most efficient and restful way to breathe. Many people with snoring and apnoea are chest-breathers; there are also substantial numbers who breathe predominantly with their diaphragm – all too often incorrectly. Please read on here even if you have previously 'learnt' diaphragm-breathing. *Correct* diaphragm-breathing is often very different in concept and practice from what people think.

A MUCH MISUNDERSTOOD MUSCLE

In the healthy breather, when the diaphragm contracts, flattens and descends during the in-breath, the contents of the upper-abdominal area bulge out a little in the solar plexus region. The diaphragm normally has a coordinated movement with the lower ribs, so at the same time there is a small outward movement of the lower ribs at the sides and the back. In other words, you get slightly bigger all the way around your body at the upper-waist level. This movement is a natural consequence of proper rib and diaphragm movement. The upper abdomen, just below the end of the breastbone, moves out naturally, passively – you don't 'do' it.

Exhalation is even more passive; it is an 'elastic' recoil of the chest wall, lungs and diaphragm. The diaphragm relaxes, it forms a dome shape again, and the lower ribs and upper-abdominal wall drop back in a little. Air passes from the lungs back through the upper airways into the atmosphere. The upper chest and lower abdomen are virtually still when a healthy breather inhales and exhales.

Did you note my use of the words slightly, small, little, still and passive in the above description of what correct diaphragm-breathing looks like?

As well as being inaudible, healthy breathing is almost invisible. Contrast this with the commonly held belief that the bigger your breath, and the larger the outward movement of your chest and abdomen, the better your breathing is. I'm sure you've also all heard these words of encouragement before too: big, deep, force, expand, push, fill, empty.

Before we move on to learning how to correctly breathe using the diaphragm, let me run through the most common faults I see. Rest assured that achieving correct diaphragm-breathing is usually quite easy – once you identify and 'undo' your bad habits, you can fairly well just let go and relax into the correct way of breathing.

Fault one: Upper-chest breathing

This is where the upper chest moves first or moves more than the diaphragm area. Using your chest and shoulder muscles to breathe 20 000 times a day can be exhausting and leave you with neck and shoulder pain.

Even if you don't chest-breathe all the time, in times of stress your breathing can fly back up there. Squint your eyes now – what do you notice when you breathe in? Now relax your eyes and take another breath. Feel the difference?

Even a rather mild form of tension like squinting can send your breathing to your upper chest! Your breathing could be compromised during the day simply by working at your computer in poor light.

Fault two: Rigid abdominal muscles

Consciously or unconsciously tensing the abdominal muscles and 'over effort' to maintain a flat stomach interferes with the movement of the diaphragm and therefore your breathing. I have seen athletes with super-tight abs and flat stomachs suffer performance anxiety, panic attacks, shortness of breath and poor endurance as a consequence of their induced upper-chest breathing pattern.

I've also found disordered breathing (and anxiety states) in people who have been working hard at improving 'core stability' but in effect have been holding in their stomachs all the time.

Sarah was a very fit but rather 'wired' 21-year-old who came to see me. Not only was she anxious, but she slept poorly and was exhausted all the time. She would get intensely nervous and 'airy' when working with her fitness trainer or doing Pilates classes. It took Sarah a few days of breathing retraining to undo the abdominal tension she had worked so hard at achieving, but she is now enjoying her fitness sessions as well as refreshing sleep.

Fault three: Reversed (paradoxical) breathing

Here, the upper abdomen moves in on inhalation and out on exhalation: the opposite of correct breathing. This may occur in some people only when they are under stress, but for some, it may be the usual way they breathe. If it does not resolve itself with the basic breathing retraining in this book, please see an experienced breathing teacher and/or a musculo-skeletal practitioner. If it is associated with breathing distress, seek medical help immediately.

Fault four: Belly puffing

This is where you actively use your abdominal muscles to push your belly area out as you breathe in. It is common to see people practising 'belly puffing' and erroneously calling it diaphragmatic or abdominal breathing. It is *not* natural and it is *not* helpful.

By pushing your abdomen out with every breath, you can end up arching your lower back and creating strain and even pain in the process. It's even worse if you're trying to do that against those tight abs that you have been working on. And you're not really increasing your lung capacity. The bottom of your lungs is about 7 cm below your nipple line. You are not getting air right down there into your belly region.

Fault five: Misunderstanding diaphragm-breathing

I use the term *diaphragm-breathing* to mean breathing correctly with the diaphragm, which means you draw in your air predominantly through diaphragm movement, but with the additional proviso that the size of the breath – and therefore the amplitude of diaphragm movement – is appropriate for the situation, be it rest, sleep or activity. The term diaphragm-breathing is, however, often associated with a deliberate increase in breath size and filling more of your lungs. At rest, the physiologically correct breath size or tidal volume is 500 ml. Our lungs have the capacity to take in considerably more – over 4000 ml extra for an adult male – and our diaphragm can move through a greater range to allow us to draw it in. So, compared to breathing your full lung capacity, normal resting breathing is *small-volume diaphragm-breathing*.

A big, 'deep' (full-capacity) breath is not appropriate unless you are doing vigorous physical exercise. The term *deep* is also confusing when applied to breathing because 'deep breathing' commonly means breathing with the diaphragm as it is *deep* within the body, and diaphragm-breathing is *deeper* than upper-chest breathing. But deep also denotes a lot of volume, as in deep water.

The term *abdominal-breathing* is again confusing. It is used to differentiate from upper-chest breathing, but it tends to imply there should be significant movement happening at or below the navel, which there will not be with a normal breath size at rest. So, in common usage, the terms *deep breathing* and *abdominal-breathing* refer to taking large in-breaths with diaphragm action and possibly some belly puffing as well, and then fully exhaling, emptying the lungs of as much air as possible. In common practice then, deep or abdominal breathing exercises are *large-volume diaphragm-breathing*.

Large-volume diaphragm-breathing exercises may have a place if you have an area of collapse (*atelectasis*) or consolidation in your lungs as may occur with pneumonia, or to re-expand your lungs after anaesthesia. But then you are practising those exercises for a 'special effect' or therapeutic purpose – you are not practising *normal* or *correct* breathing.

When you finish doing deep-breathing exercises you need to be aware of the potential consequences (for example, dizziness and shortness of breath) of consciously or unconsciously continuing to breathe too much air per breath. It is best to be mindful of restoring relaxed, gentle nose–diaphragm breathing as soon as possible after big, 'deep' breathing (and coughing).

HOW TO BREATHE CORRECTLY WITH THE DIAPHRAGM

If by now you have established regular nose-breathing and a relaxed upright posture, your diaphragm will automatically be more involved. Tension in your diaphragm may also have eased – muscle relaxation is yet another wonderful side-effect from addressing over-breathing.

The suggestions below aim to further improve diaphragm-breathing. Enjoy the practice – conscious diaphragm-breathing has a very relaxing effect on your nervous system and naturally reduces your (over) breathing.

The 'soft gold band'

As described earlier, the movement of your body as you breathe should occur at the lower end of your rib cage at the sides and back as well as in the solar plexus at the front (see Figure 16.1). It is important to develop a feel for this area – where the movement is when breathing is right.

It can help to imagine you have a 10 cm-wide band of skin all around your body just below the end of your breastbone that is gold in colour. I will refer to this band of skin as your *soft gold band*. It is like a wide, high, soft waistband (that is, it has 'give' in it). It expands as you breathe in, and falls back into place as you breathe out.

FIGURE 16.1: BREATHING USING YOUR 'SOFT GOLD BAND'

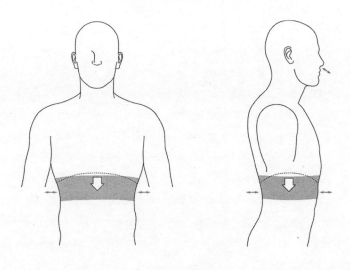

Instructions for diaphragm-breathing

Read through the following and practise each suggestion as you go, and then I will put it all together in a list – the Practice Set for diaphragm-breathing. Avoid doing the practice straight after a meal or when wearing a belt or overly tight clothing as both interfere with free diaphragm movement. Also, do not practise this when driving.

Sit with a relaxed coathanger posture, in a chair with an upright padded backrest (or use pillows to support your back). Imagine your soft gold band all around your body. As you breathe in, the gold-band area should expand slightly – that is, on the in-breath you (passively) get slightly bigger all the way around at the diaphragm level. On the out-breath the area falls back in. Can you feel this?

Relaxation of the breathing muscles is important to allow correct breathing to happen. As well as the letting go of the trunk, stomach and abdominal muscles you learnt in Chapter 14, think of your diaphragm muscle (under that soft gold band) being soft, relaxed, even 'lazy', 50 per cent made of jelly, maybe operating on four cylinders instead of eight. Then, as these muscles relax, let your breathing become lighter, simply let it happen. (Do not try to breathe to a rhythm; do not try to slow your breathing down.)

Gently, softly breathe in just the right volume of air for you and direct this air into the soft-gold-band area – front, sides, and back. Place the palm of your hand on your solar plexus. Feel for an outward movement under your hand as your gold band expands. Then, as your out-breath happens, feel the area under your hand fall back in. Just allow it to happen passively, like a balloon inflating and deflating of its own accord.

Don't force or exaggerate either movement; don't puff your abdomen out; don't tuck your stomach in; don't forcefully expel air. Simply allow the out-breath to happen; then allow the next in-breath to 'arrive' when it's ready. At the completion of breathing in, there should be no holding of the breath, but a turn and flow into the out-breath. As your breathing improves, a short automatic pause will develop at the end of the out-breath. Throughout the whole process, think of softening your stomach muscles and *letting go*.

Now, take your hand away, and while continuing to breathe 'lazily' into the soft-gold-band area, notice if you can feel outward movement in the lower side ribs, and on each side of your back in the hand-width below your shoulder blades, where your back touches the backrest of your chair. When you breathe in you should feel yourself get slightly bigger in these areas.

If you cannot feel the breath moving your back, try specifically directing the air there. Again, don't exaggerate the breath; just allow it and the movement to happen. Get your controlling self out of the way. Instead, say to yourself, 'I allow my back to be breathed' as you gently and rhythmically breathe through your nose. Allow the breath to be completely effortless; have as much air per breath and as many breaths as you need to stay completely comfortable. Closing your eyes may help.

If you feel air hunger or short of breath, this may mean you are forcing your breathing to be lighter than it wants to be at this stage. Your respiratory centre is being challenged by a higher (probably more normal) carbon dioxide level, and if the challenge is too great, this can then make you want to 'breathe up' again. You need to avoid this. Remember, have as much air as you need to stay comfortable and in control. Acclimatise at a comfortable pace.

Many people find it easier to develop relaxed diaphragm-breathing by directing the air and their attention to the movement in their back rather than the solar plexus.

Another way to help achieve this is by imagining the air that comes in through your nose going down one single pipe, which divides into two pipes, which open into each of your lungs in the area below each shoulder blade (see Figure 16.2, page 128).

When diaphragm-breathing is correctly done, you sense your breathing being lighter, while at the same time the breath is still going down into the soft-gold-band area – solar plexus, back and side ribs – even if your focus is on the back.

It's a bit like being just a little thirsty – you pour yourself a small glass of water; it just fills the bottom of the glass. Save filling your lungs to the brim for when you run up mountains.

FIGURE 16.2: BREATHING INTO YOUR BACK

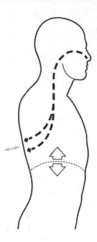

I recommend that you use your hand on your solar plexus and your back up against a padded backrest *only* in the very beginning. When you are more tuned in, you should be able to maintain diaphragm-breathing without any prompts. In fact, keeping a hand on the solar plexus can encourage active abdominal movement – puffing the belly out – which interferes with correct diaphragm action.

It is also important that you don't try to expand the soft-gold-band area by breathing in a larger volume of air than you need. Simply allow the breathing to happen in this area. Good breathing is more 'let go and allow it to happen' than 'do it this way'.

What about reducing chest movement? With relaxed diaphragm-breathing, upper chest and shoulder movement almost always gradually and naturally diminish.

PRACTICE SET: DIAPHRAGM-BREATHING

The instructions below put together all the concepts used so far for retraining good breathing. When you are doing this you are practising the first five healthy habits all at once. As before, it may help to record yourself reading these directions and then play them back when you are sitting practising until the concepts are second nature. (See the Learning resources – Audio aids to learning, page 231.)

1. Settle into the relaxed, lengthened coathanger posture.
2. Relax your jaw; have your lips together, your teeth apart.
3. Allow your body to soften and lengthen - up through your head, down through your sit bones.
4. Relax your shoulders; soften your stomach.
5. Breathe gently and smoothly through your nose.
6. Become aware of a relaxed (soft, jelly-like, lazy) diaphragm.
7. Allow your breathing to lower into the 'soft gold band'.
8. Relax and allow the gold band to expand on the in-breath.
9. Flow into the out-breath, soften your stomach muscles.
10. Breathe softly, smoothly, into the gold band.
11. Relax, let go on the out-breath.
12. Simply allow the next breath to arrive.
13. Allow your back to be gently breathed.
14. Relax, soften your stomach, let go on the out-breath.
15. Breathe as softly and smoothly as you can.
16. Practise relaxed diaphragm-breathing three to four times a day, for five to ten minutes total each time, with a short rest after five minutes.

PRACTICE TIMES

Ideal times to practise are on waking, just before bed, and one or two other times over the course of the day. You could:

- start the day either with a seated session or lying in bed on your back with your knees bent.
- do ten minutes practice before bed.
- practise while you watch TV, on the bus, waiting for a meeting, in coffee breaks, while on hold on the phone or while standing in a queue.
- lie on your left side and practise for a few minutes to help you go off to sleep.

Although you can use this technique unobtrusively anywhere, it can induce a state of significant relaxation, similar to the meditative state.

As with any sort of meditation, you should not undertake this focused diaphragm-breathing practice while driving or operating machinery.

Checking your heart rate

Check your heart rate before and one minute after a practice session, while still sitting quietly. If you have done the breathing well, your heart rate should reduce or stay the same. If your heart rate goes up by six beats or more a minute, you are likely not doing it correctly – your body is under stress.

STRATEGIES FOR DIAPHRAGM-BREATHING DURING MOVEMENT

When you are moving, your body requires more air, so it is natural to breathe more. However, poor breathers often overdo it – their breathing gets significantly faster and located more in the upper chest. This is far less efficient than a moderate increase in breathing rate and a larger tidal volume drawn in to the 'soft gold band' by a stronger movement of the diaphragm.

The principles for diaphragm-breathing during activity are the same as for sitting. I suggest you first do a focused practice session of relaxed nose–diaphragm breathing during a five-minute walk on the flat. Maintain the relaxed coathanger posture; think of free expansion of your soft-gold-band area on inhalation and the sense of allowing your back to be breathed. You will naturally draw in more air per breath to match any increased need for air. The out-breath should stay effortless, and you allow the next breath to arrive in its own time.

Once you have the concept, you can often practise nose–diaphragm breathing during your normal activities. Remember always to walk, cycle, mow and scrub only at the speed at which nose-breathing remains completely comfortable. You will likely be breathing more softly and effortlessly than you used

> **THE BIGGEST MISTAKE**
>
> The biggest mistake people make with diaphragm-breathing practice is to consciously or unconsciously increase their tidal volume and end up over-breathing. This may happen if you have been conditioned by past training to take full breaths whenever you think or hear the word 'diaphragm'. You *can* undo that conditioning.

to. Even though you may take longer to get places at first, there should be less of the breathlessness, congestion, coughing and exhaustion that came with poorly controlled breathing. Hopefully within a week or two nose–diaphragm breathing during all your activities will be your new habit and need little thought. We will take breathing control during physical exercise and sport further in Chapter 20.

ALTERNATIVE WAYS TO DIAPHRAGM BREATHE

If you have problems achieving diaphragm-breathing using these instructions, try one of the suggestions below. Note though, I have rarely needed to use them with my clients, and then for only a short period.

Half-lying position

Diaphragm-breathing may be easier for some people to achieve if they first get used to its action when lying down.

Lie on your back, with your knees bent and about shoulder width apart. Place a small support under your head. Now place your hands on your solar plexus to feel the movement – expansion as you breathe in. *Don't* expand it actively by pushing with your abdominal muscles.

The directions regarding softening and letting go of the muscles, breathing into the back, and so on, all remain the same, as they do with diaphragm-breathing in sitting. When you have got the feel for diaphragm-breathing, get up, sit in a chair, stand, or walk around and see if you can maintain it.

The diaphragm belt

What I call a *diaphragm belt* is actually an elasticised ladies fashion belt, about 8 cm wide, that does up in the front with clips. Wearing one around your upper-waist area, covering the lower ribs at the sides and over the solar plexus at the front (your soft gold band) acts as feedback for diaphragm-breathing. Choose a belt that has enough tension for you to feel the expansion of your body against it as you breathe in, but not so much tension as to be uncomfortable and restrict your breathing. Just use it until you have 'got it'.

ACTION STEPS FOR DIAPHRAGM-BREATHING

- Sit, stand and walk in the relaxed, lengthened coathanger posture.
- Breathe smoothly and gently through your nose and with your diaphragm.
- Allow your back to be *gently* breathed.
- Blend relaxed nose–diaphragm breathing into all your activities.
- Practise three or four times a day, for five to ten minute periods, until nose–diaphragm breathing is second nature.
- Check your posture and breathing once every hour (that you reasonably can).

Reassess your breathing pattern and symptoms (Tables 4.1, 4.2 and 4.3, pages 19, 26 and 30–31, respectively) after two days of diaphragm-breathing.

YOUR KEYWORDS

- Awareness
- Coathanger
- Nose
- Soften
- Soft gold band
- Let go
- Allow
- Relax and expand the band

When to move on

Move on when nose–diaphragm breathing feels habitual. If progress is slow, attention to the way you breathe during speech (Chapter 19) and your diet (Chapter 22) may help.

CHAPTER 17

Healthy habit six: Eight to twelve breaths per minute

This element of healthy breathing doesn't require specific practice because it tends to follow naturally from developing the other good habits. Your breathing automatically slows down as you change from mouth- to nose-breathing, and as you change from chest- to diaphragm-breathing. You do not need to watch a clock and practise doing eight to twelve breaths a minute. In fact, I advise against it. Deliberately breathing slower to a count may result in you compensating by breathing too heavily or too 'deeply'. It is better to simply relax into gentle diaphragm-breathing and let the timing sort itself out automatically.

How does your respiration rate now compare to normal and to what it was in Assessment 1 (Table 4.1, page 19)? If it has decreased you're on the right track. If it is above 14 and has not decreased from where it started, it looks like you need more practice of gentle diaphragm-breathing or need to investigate what is making you 'breathe up'.

Remember, your respiration rate is affected by foods you eat, medications you take, illnesses you may have, and the level of stress you are under. The average respiration rate for my clients beginning a breathing retraining program is sixteen breaths per minute. The average by day five is around eleven breaths per minute.

CHAPTER 18

Healthy habit seven: Silent, invisible breathing

For most people, when they improve their breathing through breathing retraining, there will be a reduction in both breathing rate and breath size. This naturally leads to quieter and less visible breathing.

THE SOUND OF YOUR BREATHING

Good breathing is silent. As you work at eliminating mouth-breathing and erratic and forceful breaths, airway irritation lessens, and so should your noise level when you're awake and asleep. Can you hear yourself breathing now? Can you hear yourself breathing while moving about? How does that compare to before? Have you had any comments from others about being quieter?

Now add some conscious effort to reducing any remaining noise level during the day. If your breathing is audible when doing light activities, slow down and see if it quietens while still comfortably nose-breathing. Do you need to huff and puff getting out of your chair?

INVISIBLE BREATHING

Sense how much your torso moves as you breathe. Ideally, with quiet resting breathing, there is virtually no movement seen or felt in the upper chest/collarbone/shoulder area and in the abdominal area below the navel. There is just a small movement of the soft-gold-band area – solar plexus and lower side and back ribs. Good breathing is almost invisible as well as silent.

At this stage, say three to five days into changing your breathing, if you had a high tidal volume to begin with, it is likely to be considerably less now than it was when you first picked up this book, but still likely higher than the ideal 500 ml. You are not quite perfect yet. But practice makes perfect. The best way to progress is through further relaxation while you practise diaphragm-breathing. Your breathing rate and breath size (volume) – decrease during relaxation as your need for air (oxygen) is less. You also need less oxygen as your breathing gets more efficient. You use a lot more oxygen with upper-chest breathing – those muscles are not designed for continuous usage and are very greedy for oxygen.

Remember, all exercises are to be practised with a relaxed, lengthened posture, relaxed diaphragm and shoulders, and your breathing is to remain comfortable at all times. You should not feel distressed in any way, breathless or short of air.

HIBERNATION

To move closer towards silent and invisible breathing, I use the analogy of hibernation. Hibernation is a natural physiological state in which certain animals pass the winter. It is marked by deep sleep, reduction in temperature, metabolism, heart rate and breathing rate, and a super degree of muscle relaxation. Try the following routine. (This routine also lends itself to being practised while listening to a recording of the instructions. See Learning resources – Audio aids to learning, page 231.)

Hibernation exercise instructions
PRACTICE SET: HIBERNATION
1. Sit in a comfortable chair, in the coathanger posture.
2. Allow your shoulders to soften, widen and drop.
3. Breathe smoothly and regularly through your nose.
4. Focus on relaxed, soft-gold-band diaphragm-breathing.
5. Soften your stomach muscles.
6. Allow your back to be gently breathed, then . . .
7. Pretend you are a bear sinking into hibernation, where all your body processes slow down:
    ▸ Think of your diaphragm relaxing further, moving through less distance.

- ‣ Imagine half its muscle fibres are having time off.
- ‣ Visualise the other half gradually relaxing, peacefully contracting.
- ‣ Allow your back to be more and more gently breathed, as you drift further into 'hibernation' – a fuller relaxation of all your breathing muscles – less, but enough, air per breath.
- ‣ Visualise the breathing wave pattern gradually getting smaller.
- ‣ Allow your breathing to gradually quieten.
- ‣ Allow the inhale to arrive when it's ready.
- ‣ Relax, simply let go on the out-breath.
- ‣ Breathe invisibly; breathe almost 'as if you are not breathing'.

8. Spend two to five minutes hibernating like this. Have a break for one minute and repeat.

9. If you find this comfortable, try to build up to doing five minutes continuously.

PRACTICE TIMES

Make this your way of practising your diaphragm-breathing for a total time of ten minutes, practised three to four times a day. That can be on the bus on the way to work, in quiet times before lunch and dinner, and most importantly, for ten minutes immediately before you go to bed. If you have more time available you can, if you wish, extend the total time of a practice session to twenty minutes, breaking for a short rest every five minutes.

Let me emphasise again, this technique may induce a state of very significant relaxation, similar to the meditative state and therefore, as with any sort of meditation, you should not practise it, or any form of focused relaxed diaphragm-breathing, while driving or operating machinery.

When you are comfortable and familiar with the hibernation exercise, you may extend it with the instructions below.

STILLNESS AFTER THE OUT-BREATH – THE NATURAL PAUSE

The natural and spontaneous rest point in the breathing cycle is after the exhale. Your breathing muscles and nervous system rest at this point. As your breathing improves, a short but distinct 'automatic pause' develops between the exhalation and inhalation. In a very healthy breather this natural pause may be three to four seconds. The next breath will be small, smooth and slow (see Figure 18.1).

To encourage this, see if you can experience this small relaxed 'stillness' (pause) before your next in-breath arrives. Try sitting in the stillness for a moment, before you want to breathe again. Don't grab for the next breath – let it simply 'arrive'.

FIGURE 18.1: 'HIBERNATION' AND THE NATURAL PAUSE

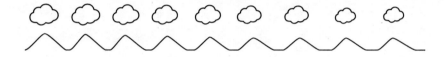

HOW DOES YOUR BREATHING FEEL NOW?

The breathing retraining instructions in the last seven chapters are aimed at bringing the rhythm, rate and volume of air that you breathe back to normal levels; to help you breathe the way you were always meant to – silently, gently, effortlessly through your nose, with a small movement at the solar plexus level, just as a healthy baby does.

If you followed all the steps correctly then you should be feeling calmer and more relaxed. Hopefully tonight you will sleep like a baby. Do you think you could snore if your breathing was slow, soft and gentle? I have lost count of the number of times I have heard this comment: 'I was breathing so quietly last night that my husband/wife had to prod me to see if I was still alive.'

If you have had decades of dysfunctional breathing, you may still feel a lot more breathing movement than I have described in these pages. Remember, you are a work in progress!

The first step is awareness of your poor breathing habits, and then step by step you gently and consistently change them. Motivation, commitment and practice are important. But if you push for too much change – reduction in breathing rate or breath size – too

SIMILARITY TO BREATHING DURING MEDITATION

People who undergo breathing retraining and achieve near perfect breathing may find that their breathing becomes almost imperceptible when they sit quietly and focus on it, and they may experience a blissful feeling of complete relaxation of mind and body – similar to that experienced during deep meditation and transcendence. It is as though the nervous system perceives the total absence of any sympathetic fight-or-flight response and switches progressively to the parasympathetic mode, with deepening relaxation of both the mind and the muscles.

People who have struggled with meditation because they have not been able to quieten the 'monkey mind' often find the meditative state easier to achieve after breathing retraining.

soon, your breathing may speed up or become uncomfortable. As always, be observant and be guided by comfort.

Check your heart rate

When you are not pushed for time, check your heart rate before practice and around a minute after you finish it. If you have done the breathing correctly, the pulse rate should reduce, or at least stay the same.

If your heart rate goes up, you are likely not relaxed and/or not breathing correctly – your body is under stress. Adjust your technique or the timing of practice as necessary – for example, not straight after a meal; not when you are hurrying to get out the door.

Also check and record your heart rate on waking each morning. As night-time and general breathing improve, it is usual to see average resting heart rates decrease and then level out into a lower range. Seeing a rise in morning heart rate can be an early indicator of illness, developing a cold, increased stress and over-breathing. Then you have an opportunity to take some measures to look after yourself. Forewarned may help you to be forearmed.

Finding your rhythm

With perfect breathing, the wave pattern is smooth and regular. The exhalation is a little longer than the inhalation. There is the natural, automatic pause of up to three to four seconds between the out-breath and the next in-breath.

If you follow the guidelines I have given for better breathing, your breathing should 'evolve' towards this ideal. As with respiration rate, you should not force your breathing into the ideal pattern – you let it find its own way there.

ACTION STEPS FOR SILENT, INVISIBLE BREATHING

- Sit in the coathanger posture.
- Breathe smoothly and gently through your nose and with your diaphragm.
- Practise *hibernating*...
- *Sit in the stillness* before the next breath.
- Breathe invisibly; breathe as if you are not breathing.
- Practise three to four times a day, for between five and twenty minutes total time each session, with a short rest every five minutes.

YOUR KEYWORDS

- Awareness
- Coathanger
- Nose
- Soften
- Soft gold band
- Let go
- Allow
- Hibernate
- Stillness

When to move on

You can move on straightaway to healthy habit eight: breathing control during speech and singing.

CHAPTER 19

Healthy habit eight: Breathing control during speech and singing

Yes, something as automatic as the way you breathe when you speak plays a role in your breathing, health and sleep equation. Improving your breathing pattern during speech can help you normalise your breathing and reduce your symptoms much faster than if you fail to tackle this issue.

PROBLEMS CAUSED BY POOR BREATHING DURING SPEECH

Talking (and singing) can make you dehydrated, breathless and congested. It can trigger coughing and tire you out. These symptoms are all precipitated or aggravated by over-breathing and difficulty coordinating breathing and talking.

Are your symptoms worse after a long day of meetings or presentations? Do you need to drink gallons when you talk a lot? If you are an over-breather, presenting to an audience can also bring on a thumping heart, sweaty palms and armpits, dizziness, nausea, going 'weak at the knees' or even going blank. These components of stage fright are well-documented symptoms of hyperventilation and acute carbon dioxide deficit!

The quick, gasping upper-chest breaths that people take during speech, generally at the beginning of a sentence, dehydrate and strain the throat. If you have a personality or a job where you talk a lot and this is the way that you speak, then you are inadvertently doing a lot of over-breathing practice. Those who need to talk a lot, like teachers, lawyers, lecturers, tour guides and salespeople, may also develop a chronic cough.

Awareness – some observations to make

To change, you need to recognise the problem – your family and friends may be more aware of gasping and breathlessness in your speech pattern than you are. Ask for their feedback. You can also try standing in front of a mirror and observing yourself as you recite a poem or tell a story. Watch for the intake of breath and whether it is through your mouth. Can you see your shoulders or chest lift? Do you notice any gasping?

You can also increase your awareness by watching and listening when others are talking and singing. See if you can spot the poor breathers on television, or when listening to talkback or songs on the radio. Notice the different breathing patterns and noises. With some people you will hear only the words; with others you will hear sharp intakes of breath. This can be particularly obvious over the phone.

GOOD BREATHING DURING SPEECH AND SINGING

It is not the lung capacity, the force and the volume of air that is important in talking and singing. Rather it is the *control* of the air. It is air passing over the vocal cords on the out-breath that makes the 'voice' and only a little air is needed to set them vibrating. The less breath you use, the better the tone. The key then is to be an efficient breather.

Australian opera singer Dame Nellie Melba wrote in her book *The Melba Method*, 'if only a little breath is necessary, it is obviously wise not to take too much air into the lungs'.[19.1] The American singer Frank Sinatra had breath control that was legendary. You could not hear him take a breath, and it was hard to see it happen.

Taking the breath in through your nose is an excellent way to control the air intake and also engages your diaphragm, which in turn controls the outflowing of air over the vocal cords. The chest and shoulders should not lift. Posture, of course, plays an important role – slouching interferes with the movement of the diaphragm.

There are many benefits of improved breathing to speech and singing, including:

- better voice projection.
- richer voice tone.

- less mucous accumulates in the back of your throat.
- less dehydration after presentations and performances.
- less fatigue at the end of a day of talking.
- greater endurance with singing.
- less breathlessness and coughing.
- remaining calm while making speeches or performing.

There is also a carry-over effect from improved control of breathing during speech – your general breathing (and snoring) and health improve at a faster rate.

STRATEGIES TO BREATHE WELL DURING SPEECH

Having already made the changes suggested in this book so far, you should now be in a better position to control your breathing during speech. The following strategies and exercises are designed to help you develop a speech-breathing pattern where you breathe in through your nose when you need air and maintain good breath control and voice projection.

When you first make these changes, you need to slow down your speech and pause momentarily, while closing your mouth, to take that next inhale through your nose. Avoid taking quick upper-chest gasps through your mouth, and speaking in such extended sentences that you become breathless.

Take the in-breaths at the natural 'punctuation' points. Your speech needs punctuation – full stops and commas, just like your writing. Punctuation in speech is a place to breathe.

Instructions – when speaking

1. Have a relaxed, upright posture.
2. Relax your jaw, throat, shoulders, breathing muscles and stomach.
3. Take the (small) in-breath through your nose.
4. Allow it into your lungs.
5. Speak slowly.
6. Shorten your sentences until you are more efficient and have better control.

7. When you need another breath, pause momentarily; close your mouth.
8. Take the next (small) in-breath silently through your nose.
9. Then continue to speak.
10. Practise by reading aloud, or doing the alphabet exercise (see below).

The alphabet exercise

This involves saying the alphabet out loud, using four gentle, silent nasal in-breaths, followed by silent, effortless breathing. Figure 19.1 shows where the pauses and in-breaths are.

The critical factors:

- All the in-breaths are small, silent, and through the nose.
- At the end of the alphabet (or sentence during normal conversation) you are gently and silently nose-breathing.
- There must be no sign of breathlessness afterwards.

FIGURE 19.1: THE ALPHABET EXERCISE

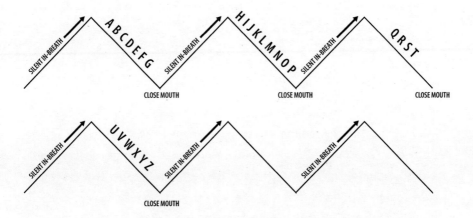

When your breathing has improved, you will be able to say the alphabet on two breaths, (A–N, and O–Z) and then later on you may get through the whole alphabet on one breath.

Your speech may be slow and somewhat stilted in the beginning. You may sound like you are delivering the Queen's Christmas message. (Interestingly, clients say that people seem to take more notice of them when they talk this way!) With practice and better breathing you become more fluent. Correct breathing is very efficient – it's hard to interrupt a good breather, as they seem to take forever to run out of breath and pause. And when they pause, it's imperceptible. Think of Frank Sinatra!

As an alternative to closing your mouth during each in-breath, you can bring your tongue into contact with the upper palate whenever you inhale. The tongue is acting like a gasket and ensuring it's a nose-breath. If you continue to have difficulty with speech, get some advice from a speech pathologist.

Singing exercise

Try singing the alphabet or the well-known 'happy birthday' song using four silent nasal in-breaths to sing the four phrases. You will see that just a small amount of air is enough to support those phrases.

TALKING AND WALKING

Until you have made significant improvements in your baseline breathing and your control during speech, it is best to not talk too much while you are exercising.

LAUGHTER

Is laughter the best medicine? Not for those who mean it when they say, 'I nearly died laughing'.

Laughter, while generally very good for us, does involve repeated extra-deep breaths and is well known to produce coughing spasms and asthma symptoms. Over 50 per cent of asthmatics report that laughter can provoke symptoms. It is important for those with breathing problems to try to maintain a level of control during laughter.

Instructions – when laughing

Take the in-breaths through your nose if you can. Between bouts of laughter, recover with nose-breathing. It may help to do a couple of short breath holds – two to three seconds, to replenish your carbon dioxide after laughing.

ACTION STEPS FOR BREATH CONTROL IN SPEECH, SINGING AND LAUGHING

- Become self-aware.
- Take the in-breaths through your nose when speaking, singing and laughing.
- Speak slowly; shorten your sentences.
- Punctuate your speech with brief pauses.
- Practise speaking or singing in front of a mirror.
- Practise the alphabet exercise or reading out loud.
- Control your breathing during and after laughing.
- Use short breath holds if necessary to recover from laughing.

CHAPTER 20

Healthy habit nine: Breathing well during exercise

Health benefits from regular exercise include an improved cardiovascular system, stronger bones, improved sensitivity of your cells to insulin, and an increase in the ability of your body to burn fat, thus offering some protection from heart disease, diabetes, osteoporosis and obesity. Exercise can also be a great stress-reliever, have an antidepressant effect, and give you a healthy dose of sunlight on your skin.

Exercise is very useful in discharging the adrenaline-mediated fight-or-flight response that is so closely tied to a pattern of over-breathing. When you are stressed and over-breathing, your body is geared up for exercise. By doing something active, even if it's just a brisk walk, you can use up some of the excess adrenaline and glucose in your bloodstream, reducing the likelihood of stress-related diseases.

Many people today are too busy or too tired to exercise, and the typical day involves little movement – drive to work, sit at a desk for eight to ten hours, drive home, sit in front of the television, and lie down in bed. We move less in a day than did our forebears, who had to chop wood, wash clothes by hand, work on the land, and walk to the markets and social gatherings.

A sedentary lifestyle and a lack of exercise can indeed be detrimental to your health. Conversely, exercise can actually exacerbate certain health problems and even bring on various symptoms and ailments. We have all heard of exercise-induced asthma and exercise-induced heart attacks. A recent internet search of 'mowing (the lawn) and heart attacks' elicited links to many articles. What was most interesting was that there were articles about the not-uncommon observation of heart attacks occurring during or after mowing, while other articles were promoting the heart attack–reducing benefits of exercise and suggested lawn mowing as one example of a healthy activity! Confusing, isn't it?

I believe that how you breathe during exercise and in the period immediately afterwards is a major factor in determining which way your experience of exercise swings.

The key to healthy exercise is to breathe well. And the master-key is nose-breathing.

Unfortunately, you can't look at the average elite athlete as an example of the best way to breathe during exercise, or at rest for that matter. Training in breathing in sports institutions is not a high priority compared to training for strength, endurance and skill. There is little emphasis placed on assessment of breathing pattern. Being at peak fitness does not necessarily mean peak health or perfect breathing.

Athletes suffer more than their fair share of respiratory illnesses. Sportspeople may also experience 'burn out', anxiety, fatigue and immune dysfunction due to pushing their bodies to the limit – most likely while breathing inefficiently. Having an Olympic gold medal does not necessarily mean you have optimal breathing. I have worked with many elite athletes and without exception they have had dysfunction-al breathing patterns at rest and during performance. Over-breathing was the rule. It is impossible to achieve optimal performance without optimal breathing.

By taking the principles of correct breathing into exercise, you can not only improve your fitness and the safety and enjoyment of exercise, but it actually helps you to improve and recondition your breathing faster. This can translate into faster reduction in symptoms, including snoring.

Do the opposite – push your breathing and blood chemistry further from normal as you exercise – and you may pay for it by worsening your baseline breathing pattern, increasing your symptoms, and maybe producing new ones.

THE TARAHUMARA RUNNERS

These legendary endurance runners from the Copper Canyon in northern Mexico traditionally breathe only through the nose. They live in a hot environment with steep canyons and run up to 120 km in a day. In fact, legend has it that the Tarahumara can run non-stop for three days and three nights. To hunt deer, they chase it on foot until the deer is exhausted. To them, running is a way of life.

The Tarahumara have been the subject of scientific study. Researchers found that on finishing a marathon (42 km), their breathing was effortless and calm; they had significantly lower heart rates than is usual, and they had lower blood pressure at the finish than at the start! They also had little need for water. What is the secret to their amazing ability that has stunned the researchers? It is said to be nose-breathing. Some indigenous peoples in Africa are also said to have had a 'culture' of nose-breathing during running.

BREATHING CHANGES DURING EXERCISE

When exercising, you do need to breathe more air than when resting. But you don't need to do it on purpose. It is not the physical activity that deepens your breathing. The activity increases your metabolism, and then breathing naturally becomes faster and deeper in line with that.

Production of carbon dioxide increases in your working muscles; more oxygen is used as 'fuel'. The increased carbon dioxide naturally stimulates breathing. The greater the intensity of exercise, the greater the metabolic rate, the greater the carbon dioxide production and the more breathing will deepen. Heart rate and blood flow also increase to deliver more oxygen to the cells and to transport more carbon dioxide to the lungs to be exhaled. Breathing naturally becomes more audible during physical exercise.

As you move, your breathing should naturally adapt so as to maintain optimal amounts of both carbon dioxide and oxygen in your blood. During prolonged intensive exercise you may breathe ten times more air per minute than at rest.

How do you know you have it right? It feels good. No stress. (And not much sweat!)

HEALTHY BREATHING DURING EXERCISE

Healthy breathing during exercise is in and out of the nose and uses the diaphragm efficiently. Inhaling through the nose ensures filtering, humidification and warming of the air. It is particularly important when exercising in dry or cold conditions. Exhaling through the nose also helps maintain hydration of the nasal tissues and sinuses. Nose-breathing during exercise is perfectly natural. It is possible and comfortable *when your baseline breathing pattern is right.*

For excellent breathers, only high-intensity exercise may require mouth-breathing – for example, during repeated 'explosive' sprints in football. Even then they quickly recover and soon switch back to relaxed nose-breathing. It's hard to find a nose-breathing runner to observe in western cultures, but check out a horse race – those majestic creatures run their heavy bodies at such speed and over such long distances, while breathing through their noses. (The jockey may have his mouth open.)

In healthy people, respiration rate should not need to go above sixteen breaths per minute during mild to moderate, continuous motion aerobic-type exercise, like brisk walking, cycling or jogging. It is better to get the increased minute volume you need through a combination of a *moderate* increase in the *number* of breaths per minute and a *significant* increase in the *amount* of air in each breath. This is achieved through proper breathing rhythm and diaphragm action. This breathing pattern is very different to what I observe in the average social exerciser and the elite athlete (see Table 20.1).

It is appropriate to breathe faster than sixteen breaths per minute during intense or maximal exertion and explosive-type exercise like sprinting, but even then the respiration rate of the healthy breather will be considerably lower than that of the poor one.

TABLE 20.1: BREATHING DURING MILD TO MODERATE EXERCISE

Healthy breathing	Poor breathing
Nose-breathing	Mouth-breathing
Diaphragm-breathing	Upper-chest breathing
16 or fewer breaths/minute	25+ breaths/minute
Quiet or moderately audible breathing	Noisy, heavy breathing

POOR BREATHING DURING EXERCISE

Dysfunctional breathing during exercise is typically through the mouth, excessively fast, and over-involves the upper-chest breathing muscles. These muscles consume a lot more energy than the diaphragm and fatigue easily. Rapid breathing also doesn't allow time to oxygenate the blood adequately and contributes to breathlessness and early fatigue.

Another fault is to forcefully exhale as much air as possible – usually through the mouth. The consequences of over-breathing during exercise may include:

- dehydration of airways
- overproduction of mucous
- less oxygen available to organs and tissues (the Bohr effect)
- angina
- asthma
- shortness of breath
- performance anxiety
- lactic acid accumulation in muscles.

After years of encouragement to breathe deeply, fully and forcefully during sports and fitness sessions, Ella found that by practising relaxed 'lower' volume diaphragm-breathing, exercise was feeling less stressful, she could exercise for longer without fatigue, and recovery was faster.

When someone who habitually over-breathes or mouth-breathes starts to exercise, their breathing will increase proportionately. Like out-of-tune cars, inefficient breathers need many more litres of fuel per kilometre than their efficient counterparts; they are noisier, and are more prone to breakdown.

Exercise professionals and amateurs alike are obsessed with the myth that taking in heaps of oxygen and pushing out as much carbon dioxide as possible on the exhalation is healthy. In fact, forced over-breathing causes blood vessels to constrict and oxygen molecules to cling tightly to the red blood cells, with the result that there is not enough oxygen available to the muscles and every-where else.

Have you noticed the distress many athletes are in, during and at the finish of events? Red in the face, sweating profusely, muscles tight and cramping, mouth wide open, suck-ing in the air but seemingly unable to get enough. (Stretcher-bearers are often on standby at the end of endur-ance events.) By contrast, the Tara-humara are observed to have a look of peacefulness on their faces and ease in their bodies after completing a long run.

> **LACTIC ACID**
>
> Lactic acid is a by-product of *anaerobic metabolism*. Metabolism is anaerobic when there is insufficient oxygen available to the muscles. A build-up of lactic acid is what makes muscles sore, tired and prone to injury. I have seen professional athletes develop lactic acid build-up symptoms within the first minute of warm-up – with what should have been mild aerobic exercise! Through breathing retraining they have been able to shift their *anaerobic threshold*, thereby delaying or even totally preventing lactic acid symptoms.

'NO PAIN, NO GAIN', OR IS IT 'TOO MUCH PAIN, ALL IN VAIN'?

Breathing incorrectly places stress on your lungs, heart and muscles during and after exercise. I have seen 'fitness fanatics' with poor breathing who look extremely unwell after an intensive cardio session at the gym. They have had very noisy breathing and bright-red faces, and some have had a repetitive cough and limped with pain (from lactic acid build-up). They might be able to complete a tough routine, but I wonder what the long-term cost might be. No amount of physical exercise on top of poor breathing is ever going to achieve robust good health.

Does it still sound impossible to jog or cycle with your mouth shut? What seems impossible now can change when you have improved your baseline breathing pattern enough.

When you are an efficient breather, you can get by comfortably with a lot less air, and the amount available with nose-breathing becomes sufficient.

BENEFITS OF BETTER BREATHING DURING EXERCISE

Frequently reported benefits following breathing retraining include:

- feeling energised rather than exhausted.

- effortless rather than restricted breathing.
- less dehydration and need for fluids.
- less need for asthma reliever medication.
- fewer stitches; less cramping and muscle soreness.
- improved speed and endurance.
- faster recovery.
- lower heart rate than usual for same intensity exercise (see Table 20.2).

TABLE 20.2: TYPICAL HEART RATE CHANGES SEEN WITH BREATHING RETRAINING

	Before	Day five
Average heart rate at rest	78	63 (19% reduction)
Average heart rate after two-minute medium pace walk	91	67 (26% reduction)

Subject to your overall health circumstances, as your breathing improves you may notice that you can go faster, tackle bigger hills or bigger players, and lift more weight at the gym. However, you need to back off somewhat on all these in the early training stage. (This can initially be hard on the ego.) With the help of an experienced teacher and a full breathing retraining program, improved performance can be achieved in as little as five days.

CARBON DIOXIDE – A PERFORMANCE-ENHANCING 'DRUG'

I have seen breathing retraining produce phenomenal improvement in social exercisers, professional athletes and Olympic champions. So dramatic have the results been at times that the athletes have been questioned by their coaches as to the source of their sudden 'performance enhancement'.

This is carbon dioxide acting like a performance-enhancing drug! It enhances oxygen delivery to the working muscles. It is not a banned substance – it is meant to show up in your bloodstream. But when exercise looks too easy, people can get suspicious.

At interschool cross-country events, parents and teachers were used to seeing the competing children red in the face, doubled up with stitches and stomach cramps, and even vomiting at the finish line. At one such event my ten-year-old son came into sight and sprinted to the finish line a good 50 m in front of the next runner. His mouth was shut; his breathing was calm and quiet. I overheard one of the teachers from another school say to our headmaster, 'That boy must have taken a shortcut' and the headmaster replied, 'No way, not this kid, but I know his mother does something funny with breathing.'

STRATEGIES FOR BREATHING WELL DURING EXERCISE

You are ready to work on improving your breathing during physical exercise if your breathing is quieter, slower and more controlled than it used to be, and you now breathe comfortably through your nose and with your diaphragm (most of the time at least), including when you are walking. If not, spend more time practising those habits or seek help from a breathing teacher.

Increasing your daily exercise can be as simple as walking to the shops, parking the car further from the office or taking the stairs rather than the lift. It is also important to find a type of exercise that you enjoy.

Begin with an activity and intensity that you are used to, and which is relaxed and rhythmical, like walking, riding a stationary exercise bike or jogging. Start on the flat.

Be led by your nose

Let your nose dictate the pace of your exercise. That is, don't exercise to the point where you have to open your mouth. As you improve you can gradually increase your pace, distance or the gradient.

If your nose starts to block up or drip, or you begin to puff or feel breathless, then you are moving too fast for your current breathing status. Your breathing fitness is not yet up to your leg fitness.

Let's think of the golden rule again: *Go only as fast as your nose will comfortably allow.*

And we can add to it: *Go slow now to be faster later.*

Maintain coathanger posture and use your diaphragm well

Exercise as though you have your coathanger in position, relaxing and dropping your shoulders, lengthening your body upwards through your head as you are moving forwards – walking/running tall.

As you do this, your breathing eases and centres on your diaphragm. By keeping your stomach muscles relaxed, your diaphragm can move freely, adapting to any increased requirements for air.

As you go up a hill, it moves through a larger amplitude, naturally drawing in more air per breath. This also allows your ribs to move as nature intended. Your whole soft-gold-band area will expand more. Tell yourself, 'relax and expand the band'.

For the out-breath, as always, let it be passive. Think of the exhalation simply *falling out* and the next breath arriving in its own time. Relax into your natural rhythm.

When you go downhill, your air requirement reduces, and so will your (lower) chest expansion.

Correct use of the diaphragm will mean there is little upper-chest involvement in mild and moderate intensity exercise. (A diaphragm belt may be helpful initially as a guide to where torso expansion should be, see page 131.)

The golden rule here is: *The more intense the exercise, the more your soft gold band expands* (see Figure 20.1).

FIGURE 20.1: BREATHING DURING EXERCISE

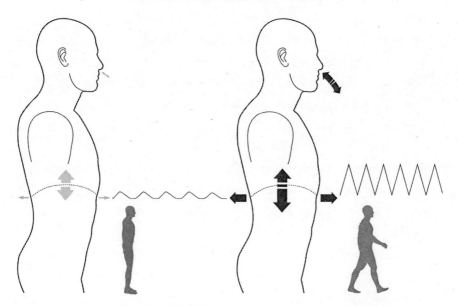

Respiration rate of sixteen or less

Your respiration rate at rest and during exercise naturally tends to be less with diaphragm-breathing than with upper-chest breathing. In my experience, having a breathing rate of sixteen breaths or less per minute during mild to moderate aerobic-type exercise (training-pace not racing-pace) is efficient and promotes improvement in your fitness, performance and breathing. Slower, deeper/fuller breathing during exercise is more efficient and comfortable than faster, more shallow upper-chest breathing.

To check your breathing rate, first have steady and gentle nose–diaphragm breathing happening while you walk or jog at a comfortable pace on the flat. Then count your in-breaths for one minute, using a watch or stopwatch while you keep moving.

If your rate is sixteen or less it is helpful then to determine the rhythm where your steps comfortably synchronise with your breathing (see Figure 20.2, page 156). For example, you may find that when you walk breathing comfortably at fifteen breaths a minute, you take three steps during the in-breath, and three steps during the out-breath; someone else may do three on the in-breath, four on the out-breath.

Someone who is fitter and breathes well may walk considerably faster, take fourteen breaths per minute and take five steps on the in-breath and five steps over the out-breath. (There are no strict rules here as there are so many variables to consider.) Use this information as a guide to help you work out your body's comfortable, natural breath–step rhythm. Then you no longer need to count or refer to a stopwatch as you will naturally fall into this pace.

If your breathing rate is more than sixteen breaths per minute, or if you feel you are not getting enough air, you (your legs) may be going too fast for your current breathing-fitness level. Slow down both your leg pace and your breathing pace a bit to see if you can find a comfortable rhythm.

Allow yourself as much air per breath as you need to satisfy yourself. Remember, it's individual. These are guidelines only; find your own comfortable pace.

The golden rule here is: *Stay comfortable and in control.*

FIGURE 20.2: A 3/4 BREATH-STEP RHYTHM

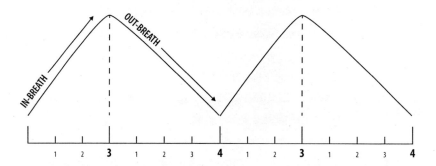

Bronwyn had been fitness training on the same hill for years, always getting aches in her legs within five minutes of starting up the hill. Using her diaphragm properly and keeping her respiration rate below sixteen breaths saw the end of the aching legs.

Recovery

After a 'warm down' recovery period, spend five minutes focusing on comfortable, relaxed nose–diaphragm breathing. Your breathing rate will gradually decrease to your resting rate. This will also help bring your heart rate back towards resting rate.

PRACTICE SET: NOSE–DIAPHRAGM BREATHING DURING EXERCISE

1. Choose a mild to moderate aerobic and continuous-motion type exercise.
2. Practice relaxed nose–diaphragm breathing for two minutes before starting .
3. Start out at a slower pace (initially).
4. Maintain the relaxed, lengthened coathanger posture.
5. Breathe in and out through your nose.
6. Breathe with a relaxed diaphragm motion.
7. Have a soft stomach.
8. Allow the soft-gold-band/diaphragm area to expand on the in-breath.
9. Allow your back to be breathed.
10. Let go on the out-breath.
11. Allow deeper, fuller breaths as your need increases.
12. Allow yourself to have all the air you need.
13. Aim to breathe no more than sixteen breaths/minute for mild–moderate exertion.
14. Find your natural rhythm for breathing and stepping.
15. Do not strain.
16. Gradually increase your pace/gradient as your comfort allows.
17. Control your breathing during warm down and recovery.
18. Practise relaxed nose–diaphragm breathing for five minutes after warm down.

PRACTICE TIMES

Build up gradually to a total of 30 minutes exercise a day, four to six times per week if appropriate. (You can start as low as a trip to the letterbox and back.) The 30 minutes does not have to be done in one go.

Note: When your aim is to improve your breathing pattern, it is best to immediately reduce your pace, or stop, the moment you feel any symptoms or indications of pain or discomfort, rather than pushing yourself to the point where you have to open your mouth to breathe.

Of course, it is a different situation if you are aiming to win a medal or a premiership.

Remember: *Comfortable and in control.*

Inadequate noses

Some people may have noses that are simply too narrow to allow sufficient air intake during physical exercise. This could be caused by congenital defects, poor skeletal development and/or the effects of chronic mouth-breathing. However, everyone's breathing can be improved to some extent. Mouth-breathing can become more efficient and controlled.

A special note on swimming

Yes, you can breathe through your nose while swimming. It requires healthy baseline breathing (resting minute volume 4–6 litres/min), good breath awareness, and a refined breathing/stroke technique with good control and timing. This may be difficult to achieve without individual coaching.

However, once you have more efficient breathing on land, you will need less air-as-fuel when you swim, just as when you run. So the in-breaths you take when swimming, even if through your mouth, can be smaller than they used to be and just as, if not more, comfortable.

What some people have found after breathing training is that instead of taking a breath with every second or third freestyle stroke, they can easily take fewer breaths, for example breathing (albeit through the mouth) every fourth or fifth stroke.

MAKING PROGRESS

Increase your speed, distance and the incline gradually as your breathing and fitness improve. Heart and muscle function are very dependent on blood and oxygen supply, so getting your breathing right is the essential first step to improving your health and fitness.

When you first exercise with nose-breathing, it can be difficult to keep pace with someone else or carry on a conversation. Either walk alone until you have your rhythm and control or let the other person know that you won't be as fast or chatty as usual. Otherwise you could find yourself mouth-breathing and hyperventilating.

Once you have your 'nose–diaphragm rhythm' you can try other forms of exercise like rowing, gardening or dancing; then the less rhythmic forms like tennis.

If you have been exercising with your mouth open all your life, as is the case for most people, then you are going to have some unlearning and reconditioning to do. Eventually nose–diaphragm breathing can be the norm.

> My youngest son had been joining me on an early morning run from the age of five. He had only ever known nose-breathing when running. At the age of twelve he started at a new school. The sports teacher was watching 'the new talent' during the various events at the athletics carnival. Tom had already won the 100, 200 and 400 m races. Now he was running the 1500 m. As he effortlessly ran the laps of the oval, the sports teacher must have thought Tom was not really trying, not giving his all. He looked too laid-back compared to the other boys who were 'really' trying – gulping for air, red in the face, or struggling with a stitch. As Tom passed him on the final laps, the teacher yelled out, 'open your mouth'. Tom didn't. He won the race easily.
>
> I knew the teacher's instruction would have been very embarrassing and disconcerting for my son. I said to him afterwards that I hoped he hadn't ignored the teacher just because he knew I was watching. Tom's response was 'No, I tried to open my mouth but I just couldn't work out how to do it'.

It is important to get the nose–diaphragm breathing regime to be like second nature during low intensity exercise, before you adapt it into intensive or competitive exercise. Breath size and rate both need to increase as intensity increases. When you have physiologically normal breathing your nose can cope with a substantial further increase in both. You can generally improve more rapidly if you do an intensive breathing retraining program with a teacher.

ADVANCED TRAINING

The work I do with athletes begins the same as with anyone else – they improve their baseline breathing first. Then they apply the principles during activity, then while walking, and then jogging, running, cycling, rowing, swimming, and so on. After four days on an intensive breathing retraining course, athletes are usually ready to apply more advanced breathing techniques during training at the gym, field, track or pool, and with more vigorous physical exertion. I was never surprised when they called me to report personal bests less than two weeks later.

That said, such intensive, individualised, guided and fine-tuned training, and the targeted application for specific sports, is unfortunately beyond the scope of this book.

FINAL THOUGHTS ON PHYSICAL ACTIVITY

Unfortunately, these days few people breathe correctly sitting in a chair or sleeping, let alone when exercising. You only have to observe how many people need to have their mouth open simply to stroll through the mall – and this is not vigorous exercise with high oxygen demands.

The fact that most people breathe through their mouth when exercising does not mean it is normal. We are meant to be nose-breathers, so let us live, sleep and move as nature intended.

ACTION STEPS FOR BREATHING WELL DURING EXERCISE AND SPORT

- Introduce nose–diaphragm breathing into an aerobic exercise routine.
- Go slower initially.
- Gradually increase your pace as your breathing improves.
- Pace yourself to breathe no more than sixteen breaths/minute for mild–moderate exertion.
- Control your breathing during warm down and recovery.

YOUR KEYWORDS FOR EXERCISE

- Awareness
- Coathanger
- Nose
- Soft stomach
- Soft gold band
- Let go
- Allow
- In over ... steps, out over ... steps

THE GOLDEN RULES:

Go only as fast as your nose will comfortably allow.

Go slow now to be faster later.

The more intense the exercise, the more your soft gold band expands.

Comfortable and in control.

Too much pain, all in vain.

CHAPTER 21

Strategies for panic attacks, colds and insomnia

Disturbed breathing is an obvious feature during panic attacks and with colds. Though less obvious with insomnia, disturbed breathing can be contributing to a hyper-arousal state that prevents sleep. Improving your breathing can make a big difference in preventing these conditions. In addition, there are some useful strategies you can apply to help manage them.

A panic attack is a sudden surge of overwhelming anxiety and fear. Your breathing speeds up, your heart pounds, you may be dizzy or nauseated or feel 'spaced out', and you may find it difficult to breathe.

Panic attacks can, among other things, be a response to stressful or dangerous situations or to anxiety. Sometimes the panicky breathing can seem to appear out of the blue, or you can wake with it from a bad dream or following an apnoea episode.

While it is important to identify and address the cause of panic attacks, the better your baseline breathing pattern, the less likely you are to flip into panicky breathing. Even if you cannot eliminate all the stresses in your world, you can change your body's response.

In the case of head colds, becoming a gentle nose-breather confers protection against airborne infective particles and helps maintain moist mucous membranes.

In terms of insomnia prevention, improving your breathing can decrease your level of physiological arousal and facilitate the relaxation response.

PANIC ATTACKS

A great strategy to help manage panic attacks is to do a sequence of short breath holds (see page 99). These can also be helpful if you have a cold or insomnia, or you need help with emotional shock, stage fright or waking suddenly with a racing heart. The short breath holds address hyperventilation and calm down panicky breathing and a revved-up nervous system. They can be used anywhere and anytime and require no equipment.

The sequence of short breath holds is used to gently raise carbon dioxide which can:

- interrupt a pattern of erratic or rapid breathing.
- stabilise airway mast cells and prevent histamine release.
- reduce nasal congestion and inflammation.
- slow and calm breathing.
- deactivate the fight-or-flight response and calm you.

Instructions

1. Pause your breath for one or two seconds.
2. Breathe again, in and out, in and out . . . (as slowly and gently as you comfortably can) for about three to four breaths (fifteen to twenty seconds).
3. Repeat steps 1 and 2 until relief is felt or for five minutes, whichever comes first (see Figure 21.1A).
4. As your breathing eases, you can progress from pauses of one second to two seconds and then to three seconds. You can work the pattern up, then back down again, repeating each stage twice. Do this for five to ten minutes (see Figure 21.1B).

As always, with the short breath holds, you must avoid pausing your breath for a length of time that provokes a larger inhalation afterwards or any breathlessness. This is counterproductive.

Don't repeat the sequence of short breath holds too quickly – allow at least three breaths in between each pause.

FIGURE 21.1: SHORT BREATH HOLD SEQUENCE – TWO LEVELS

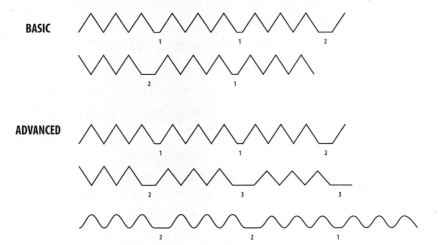

My clients have found the short breath hold sequence to be very helpful in calming themselves in situations of acute stress, anxiety, panic or breathlessness or when experiencing uncomfortable symptoms like gasping breathing, a racing heart or sweaty palms.

In an acute situation like a panic attack, initially just focus on slowing down your breathing by introducing the small pauses. Don't worry at first about nose-breathing, good posture and your diaphragm – once you are feeling calmer you can give them attention.

While it is best to use the pauses with nose-breathing, they can still be helpful with mouth-breathing, or a combination of the two. You can pause your breathing anywhere in the cycle, although it is preferable after the exhale. Take medication as necessary and as advised by your doctor.

ACTION STEPS FOR RELIEF OF PANIC BREATHING

- Practise the short breath hold sequence for five minutes, twice a day, for three days to familiarise yourself with it. (Then you have it at the ready should a situation arise.)
- Use the short breath hold sequence for five to ten minutes to calm your breathing in a panic situation.

- Use the hibernation exercise instead if it works better for you (see page 135).
- Address any psychological or medical issues that underlie your condition.
- Avoid foods and drinks that elevate your breathing rate (see Chapter 22).
- Try to maintain good breathing for long-term control and prevention.

> I had not yet met Mia but I had spoken to her a few days earlier when she had phoned to book a consultation. When she called again she was very distressed and asked to speak to me. Over the phone I could hear her rapid, heavy breaths and the panic in her voice. She was not only distressed but dizzy and confused. No time for explanations, I asked her to simply follow my voice, and told her that I would check with her soon about how she was doing. I told her I would introduce short pauses into her breathing with the words, 'Pause one, two' (about one second to start with). I listened for the ins and outs of Mia's breathing and introduced the short pauses every three to five breaths. After about eight cycles, I could no longer hear her breathing and I added, 'Now try to breathe through your nose if you have not already switched over to it. Breathe as softly as you can . . . Now, how are you feeling?' The answer was, 'Amazing'. Mia said that she felt completely calm, her heart had stopped thumping and her armpits were no longer dripping. Even I was amazed at the power of the short breath hold sequence and yet I had seen many times before the look of wonder and relief on people's faces after coaching them through panic attacks.

COLDS

Breathing rates naturally elevate during fever or infection. If you already have baseline over-breathing, a further rise in breathing rate can mean increased intensity of your symptoms.

As the airways narrow with inflammation and congestion and your volume of breathing increases, then louder snoring, more apnoea, and greater fatigue are likely. Anything you can do to calm and control your breathing may help you reduce symptoms and overcome the acute illness faster.

Strategies include side-sleeping, elevating the head end of the bed and avoiding over-sleeping. Also avoid foods and drinks that increase your breathing rate – they will elevate your nasal congestion and mucous production.

For most people, the worst culprits are strong tea, coffee, milk, and high-starch/high-sugar foods. You should always favour light and cleansing foods. A slice of chocolate cake with ice-cream may taste great but you might end up wondering whether it was worth the cost, as it is more likely to be followed by a blocked nose than a snack consisting of fruit and nuts.

Even with a cold, you should still breathe as much as possible through your nose, even though it is more difficult. You may find five to ten minutes practice of the short breath hold sequence helpful in relieving congestion. Try it several times during the day and just before bed. Taking the time to review the suggestions in Chapters 13 (Nose-breathing) and 22 (Food–breathing connection) may help.

If the strategies here do not relieve your congestion enough, you may have to resort to mouth-breathing for a time. If you find yourself in that situation, be mindful to breathe as gently through your mouth as you can. Try the short breath hold sequence from time to time and check every now and again to see if your nose is now clear enough to breathe through.

Yes, even mouth-breathing can be done in a better way. *Volume control* is one of the most important elements in improving breathing, and you can do that with mouth-breathing. Don't, however, allow yourself to slip back into mindless larger volume mouth-breathing and undo some of your good progress.

Take care with nose blowing – only blow if necessary, and then as gently as you can. Follow nose blowing with a short breath hold of one to three seconds. Forceful nose blowing can cause sinus and ear problems.

In my experience, people who have successfully normalised their breathing usually find that colds become less frequent and of shorter duration.

Jackie had asthma and she also snored. She got frequent colds that would go to her chest every time, resulting in increased asthma symptoms and bronchitis. Anything that was going around the office, you could be sure that Jackie would get it first, come down with it hardest, and be off work for longer than anyone else. At a six-month follow-up after a breathing retraining course Jackie very excitedly told me that she had just gone through a whole winter without having a day off work. The first cold she caught had just stayed in her nose and there was no sign of asthma. The next cold that struck her office wiped out everyone else but left her untouched.

ACTION STEPS FOR DEALING WITH A COLD

- Try to nose-breathe as much as possible – slow down activities if necessary.
- Avoid strenuous activity that makes you mouth-breathe.
- Avoid known allergens or trigger factors.
- Try five to ten minutes practice of the short breath hold sequence for relief of nasal congestion.
- If you have to mouth-breathe as your nose is so blocked, make it as gentle as you can.
- Rest more but don't sleep more than usual.
- Recline rather than lie down to rest, if possible, during the day.
- Elevate the head end of the bed at night.
- Avoid strong tea and coffee.
- Don't overeat.
- Avoid those foods and drinks that increase your breathing rate.
- Consider the use of a saline nasal spray.
- See your doctor if you have a high temperature, a lung disease or sudden weakness.

INSOMNIA

By controlling your breathing you can make use of carbon dioxide's sedative effects on the body. Inducing a slight rise in carbon dioxide by calming your breathing down before sleep may reduce excessive brain activity and help to reduce insomnia and nightmares.

Many clients have successfully used the short breath hold sequence while lying in bed to get off to sleep (see Figure 21.1B). They tell me it works better than counting sheep. It's portable too – you don't have to remember to pack it when travelling. Even just the practice of gentle diaphragm-breathing as you lie in bed may be sufficient.

The short breath hold sequence can also be used if you wake up in fright from apnoea or a dream or if you wake up and can't get back to sleep. Think of it as deactivating your fight-or-flight response or like taking a natural sedative.

In addition to general improvement in your breathing and use of the short breath hold sequence, developing good sleep habits (*sleep hygiene*) can be very helpful.

Regular aerobic exercise, like walking, has been found to promote a better sleeping pattern. Make sure you do it with comfortable nose-breathing. It is best not to exercise too close to sleep time – early morning exercise or three to four hours before bed seems to be most conducive to sleep. If you are outside walking, then you can also be getting some sunshine.

Also be aware that an overly warm bedroom temperature or too many bedclothes can cause your body to over-heat, leading to over-breathing and poor sleep. It will also interfere with the natural drop in body temperature that is associated with sleep.

Lastly, insomnia may be related to various health conditions and medications, and it is important to be checked for conditions

> **GOOD SLEEP HABITS**
> - Relaxation of an evening.
> - Avoiding work, exercise, worry or stimulating activities of an evening (no horror movies!).
> - Dimming the lights in your home in the evening.
> - Not eating within two to three hours before going to bed.
> - Avoiding foods that stimulate you or increase your breathing (Chapter 22).
> - Not drinking alcoholic or caffeinated drinks of an evening.
> - Taking a warm shower or bath two hours before bedtime.
> - Going to bed around the same time each evening.
> - Getting up at the same time every day.
> - Keeping the use of sleeping pills for short-term purposes only (if at all).
> - Having a bedtime ritual.
> - Keeping a sleep diary.

underlying chronic insomnia. For example, anxiety and depression can be serious conditions that may be accompanied by insomnia. People with such conditions should be under the care of a doctor. Similarly, people whose insomnia may be related to alcohol or drug addiction should also seek help to manage these difficult issues.

ACTION STEPS FOR INSOMNIA RELIEF

- Develop good sleep habits.
- Exercise regularly, but not within three hours of bedtime.
- Avoid over-heating in bed.
- Do ten minutes of relaxed diaphragm-breathing practice before bed.
- Try the short breath hold sequence for five to ten minutes if you have trouble getting to sleep.
- Address any psychological or medical issues that underlie your insomnia.
- Avoid foods and drinks that elevate your breathing rate.
- Normalise your breathing for the long term.

CHAPTER 22

The food–breathing connection

In Chapter 8 we looked at the reasons why people develop bad breathing habits. Food choices, together with eating practices, can be a contributory factor in over-breathing. In this chapter we will look at ways in which you can support better breathing by making healthier choices in how, when and what you eat.

Many people find their breathing responds well to retraining without having to make too many dietary changes, though, of course, good dietary choices and habits are preferable on many counts, not only in relation to breathing. Some people, however, find some additional dietary changes make a big difference in the progress they make. If you've had trouble conquering the mouth-breathing and/or fast, upper-chest breathing habits, making some changes to how and what you eat may give you just the boost you need. I will provide some pointers that my clients have found helpful as well as some general information that you may find relevant and interesting.

This chapter provides information and a discussion of dietary habits and particular foods and food combinations that may impact your breathing. It is not a diet or a full nutrition plan.

The information contained here needs to be considered in relation to individual medical conditions and your particular dietary requirements. I advise you to educate yourself widely on this topic and to discuss this information with your doctor or nutritionist before making any dietary changes.

Let's begin with a review of how breathing affects the digestion of food so that you will be able to take note of any changes in this area.

BREATHING AND DIGESTION

Earlier (Chapter 6) we looked at the many ways that incorrect breathing can have a negative impact upon various body systems. In the gastrointestinal area, over-breathing often causes digestive discomfort and dysfunction. It can contribute to dry mouth, difficulty swallowing, heartburn, colic, irritable bowel, belching, bloating, constipation and flatulence. Many of these symptoms are related to smooth muscle spasm in the gut walls. (They may also have other medical causes so check with your doctor if problems persist.)

Additionally, over-breathing causes the blood supply to the gastrointestinal tract to be reduced, compromising the process of digestion. With poor digestion the body is limited in its capacity to extract nutrients from our food and effectively use them to maintain robust health and vitality. Over-breathing also affects blood sugar metabolism, the body's acid–alkaline balance and its electrolyte balance.

Improved breathing helps to normalise metabolic processes, to increase blood flow to the gastrointestinal tract and to help the gut to function smoothly, thereby playing a pivotal role in reducing gastrointestinal problems and improving digestion. A more efficient digestive system can also translate into reduced appetite.

Many people notice improvements in digestion and energy levels within 24 to 48 hours of commencing breathing retraining. Those on a weight-loss program often find they are less hungry and results come easier. To sum up, commonly reported benefits from breathing retraining include:

- reduced constipation and flatulence
- reduction in colic and irritable bowel symptoms
- reduced heartburn
- reduction in excess appetite
- fewer cravings for processed and sugary food
- easier weight normalisation
- increased energy, exercise capacity and endurance.

Have you noticed any of these changes since working on the nine healthy breathing habits?

When you reduce over-breathing, you reduce smooth muscle spasm. This will generally make heartburn and colic less likely. However, any persistent digestive symptoms need medical attention as some other serious conditions can masquerade as symptoms like heartburn. It may also be helpful to check whether you have adequate levels of stomach acid and digestive enzymes. Both are essential for proper digestion and can be deficient, especially as we get older.

Now we will look at the flip side – how eating affects breathing. Both *how* we eat and *what* we eat have the potential to be detrimental to our breathing.

EATING HABITS THAT DISTURB BREATHING

There are four main eating habits that can disturb your breathing.

Eating when not hungry

Eating when you are not hungry can cause considerable stress to your body. When your body has to use energy to process food it does not need, your breathing increases and your digestion can be compromised.

Hunger is usually a physiological sign that your body is in need of nutrients and is ready to receive and digest food. Appetite, by contrast, is often tied up with a craving for food that is stimulated by the senses, or by thoughts and emotions. For example, you may want to eat because of an enticing aroma (like when you smell onions or bacon cooking), or as a comfort because you are upset, tired or bored. You may eat just because food is offered to you or because the clock says it is morning-tea time. You may also keep eating beyond what you need because you were trained to eat everything on your plate.

Set meal times and set quantities of food may or may not match your natural hunger cycle or your level of activity and requirement for food.

The first strategy to adopt is to listen to your body's signals to identify when you're actually hungry. That is, eat and drink according to need rather than according to etiquette, social pressure, habit and convenience.

This will have the least impact on your breathing, and will ensure the best results for digestion. Eating when hungry is more likely to correspond with the full complement of digestive juices being available for good digestion. Of course, sharing meals with family and friends is an important social activity. By getting to know your body well, you can eventually time your natural hunger to fit in with planned meal times.

Overeating and being overweight

It is estimated that we now eat between two and three times as much as we did 50 years ago, and we get far less exercise. Overeating puts stress on your body and deepens your breathing – you now know what trouble that can get you into.

If overeating also results in you becoming overweight, the extra weight you carry requires more effort and therefore more breathing for you to move around. Life becomes so much harder than it needs to be. You may have noticed overweight friends or colleagues with heavier breathing than those with normal weight. They are also more likely to snore at night, feel less energetic and be less inclined to exercise.

Many people notice that as their breathing improves, they require less food to satisfy their hunger and energy needs and they find they have more energy. Overall, they usually feel better, find it easier to exercise and can more easily shed excess weight. For the sake of your breathing and your health, tune in, eat only when hungry and stop when you've had enough.

Air gulping when eating

This can lead to shortness of breath, noisy eating and wind problems. To avoid gulping air, don't breathe in while you are actually putting food (or liquids) into your mouth.

Once the food is in, close your mouth and try to breathe through your nose while you chew and swallow. This usually results in taking smaller mouthfuls, eating and drinking more slowly, and has the additional benefit of giving your body a chance to recognise when your stomach is full.

Eating within two hours of bedtime

Increased breathing is a natural consequence of digestion. So if you have baseline over-breathing and you are still digesting when you go to bed, your breathing volume will increase further, making it even more likely you will snore. Due to the large pressure swings that go with high-volume breaths, you can even vacuum up some of the acid from your working stomach and you may well wake with heartburn.

Sitting down to eat and allowing at least two hours for digestion before bed is helpful. Allow three hours if it is a heavy meal.

'STRESSFUL' FOODS – FOODS THAT ADVERSELY AFFECT BREATHING

Increasingly, since the 1950s, we have seen a shift away from eating fresh, whole, natural plant and animal foods to a diet now dominant in highly processed man-made foods. Today we eat lots of things we are not designed to eat, and may at the same time starve ourselves of essential nutrients. We end up with bodies that do not function as they are meant to. Breathing is one of the functions that gets disturbed.

The aim of this section is to draw attention to the hazards of some of our modern-day food choices; to encourage you to make choices that will support good breathing and ultimately your health and vitality in both the short and the long term. The Appendix provides suggestions for further reading.

Prior to the industrial revolution the leading causes of death were infection and trauma, but fast-forward to today and we see that chronic degenerative diseases, or what are called 'lifestyle diseases', are now the leading cause of death in developed countries. At the top of the list are cardiovascular disease, cancer, chronic respiratory disease and diabetes. The food we eat is a major contributing factor.

The modern western 'industrialised' diet is characteristically high in processed starch- and sugar-rich foods and their assorted food chemicals. Natural animal fats have largely been replaced with highly processed, chemically altered vegetable oils and fats, while the heavy use of pesticides and other chemicals permeates food production. Along with the ascendancy of the processed diet has come a corresponding increase in the incidence of chronic degenerative diseases and mental health conditions.

We can witness this same phenomenon occurring in non-western countries. Fundamental changes in diet are taking place as these nations embrace industrial agriculture and food processing technologies. They too are recording rising rates of chronic degenerative diseases. We are also seeing lifestyle diseases showing up at younger ages. With this in mind, let's consider the following information.

Nutrient-deficient foods

This is our first category of potentially 'stressful' foods. When our diet is deficient in nutrients, our body enters a state of stress. The stress response includes increased breathing.

Unfortunately, the nutrient content of a lot of food today is likely to be deficient. A large proportion of our fruit, vegetable and grain crops are grown in soils lacking in many essential minerals and trace elements.

Many of the animals that provide a source of primary protein, healthy nutrient-dense fats, and other concentrated nutrients are not always reared on their natural food sources and this changes the quantity and quality of nutrients available. For example, red meat is normally a concentrated source of minerals because the animals spend their lives on pasture, chomping down masses of green grass and other plant matter. Today, however, cattle may spend their lives in feedlots and be grain-fed.

Further nutrients are lost from our food during storage and transportation, and can be destroyed, degraded or altered during commercial processing. Adding synthetic vitamins and minerals to processed foods just cannot compare with the synergistic array of vitamins, minerals, enzymes and antioxidants available from fresh, whole plant and animal produce, particularly when it is grown organically in nutrient-dense soils and pastures.

On a modern highly processed diet we are likely to be over-fed yet under-nourished.

Processed 'foods'

The consumption of highly processed foods comes with the potential to put a heavy metabolic and toxic load on your body. Our bodies have to work harder to digest and process unnatural foodstuffs. An increase in breathing rate is one of the first indicators of a body under stress.

Much of our food today has been grown with the use of man-made chemical products like fungicides, herbicides, pesticides, antibiotics and hormones. Further chemicals may be used during storage and transport and residues from these can be present in and on the foods as they reach our tables. Processed and manufactured foods may contain mould inhibitors, stabilisers, artificial sweeteners, preservatives to increase shelf life, and additives to colour the food and enhance flavour. Some ingredients may be genetically modified, molecularly transformed, irradiated and, frankly, fake. The list of ingredients on many packaged foods reads like an extract from a chemist's textbook. We need to be suspicious of unpronounceable ingredients and of food products that can sit on a pantry shelf for weeks, months or years and still look the same. Further contamination of our food can come from metals, phthalate (plasticiser) and plastic leaching into the food from containers and wrappings.

As well as the unhealthy substances that find their way into processed foods, the actual manufacturing processes involved – such as heating foods to high temperatures (vegetable oils and cow's milk are just two examples) or subjecting food to high pressures – damage naturally occurring fats and oils, alter the chemical structure of the food, and destroy and deplete important enzymes and nutrients. This fundamental change in the nature of food poses potential problems for our digestion and, ultimately, proper cell function as the body tries to deal with 'foreign' substances, including 'foreign' fats. Once again that message: stress your body and you stress your breathing.

Highly processed vegetable oils are commonly used in fast food, restaurants and home cooking, in margarines and dressings, and are in almost all processed foods and commercially baked goods including biscuits, pastries, cakes, crackers, breads, and some snack foods.

Processed milk and dairy products

These are known offenders or key suspects in breathing disturbance. The processing of milk greatly diminishes its nutritional value and renders it indigestible for many people. Pasteurised milk is more or less rendered 'dead' as high-temperature *pasteurisation* not only kills any harmful bacteria but also destroys the beneficial bacteria and valuable enzymes that help us to digest milk. It also diminishes vitamin content, destroys vitamin B12 and alters the structure of fragile milk proteins. The *homogenisation* process denatures the butterfat globules. Commonly reported symptoms from consumption of commercially processed milk include nasal and sinus congestion, mucous at the back of the throat, asthma and digestive upset.

Milk alternatives such as soy milk, oat milk, and rice milk are also highly processed (even more so if 'long life') and may contain preservatives and additives. These are hardly natural foods, although many people have used them without apparent problems.

I have seen the withdrawal of soy milk and commercial cow's milk from the diet dramatically improve nasal congestion in both children and adults. Over recent decades, dairy products have been relied upon for dietary calcium but nutritionists can advise on many other good sources if needed.

Poorly prepared foods

Grains, seeds and legumes need proper preparation to make them more digestible. Our healthy ancestors knew how to prepare foods for better digestion using soaking, sour leavening and fermenting. Modern food preparation often skips or shortens these important steps, sacrificing quality nutrition and digestion for speed. Your breathing may well feel the stress.

Properly fermented foods, like sauerkraut and kefir, supply your body with enzymes and friendly health-promoting bacteria. Including them in your meals allows the body to more easily digest food and at the same time supports your immune system.

Caffeinated foods: coffee, tea, cola, chocolate

Foods containing caffeine have a stimulant effect on the adrenal glands and subsequently on breathing. In excess they are detrimental to good breathing and quality sleep.

Alcohol

Alcohol can at first give you a feeling of general relaxation, including relaxed (reduced) breathing, and should you go to bed then, make it easier to fall asleep. But later, as the alcohol is metabolised, breathing deepens, with snoring, headache, agitation and/or nausea becoming a possibility. As alcohol also relaxes the throat muscles, the likelihood of airway collapse and apnoea will be even greater.

Foods that cause a spike in blood sugar

Fluctuating blood-sugar levels can stimulate your breathing. Carbohydrate foods ultimately break down to a simple sugar that is absorbed into the bloodstream.

The foods that are predominantly carbohydrate include sugar, fruit, non-starchy vegetables (e.g., green vegetables, salad vegetables), starchy vegetables (e.g., potatoes, corn) and grains (e.g., wheat, rice, oats, rye). The rate at which the carbohydrate content of these foods converts to sugar and enters the bloodstream varies. It depends on the ratio of carbohydrate to protein and fat in a given meal or snack.

A meal or snack overabundant in the more sugary and starchy carbohydrates, especially the more refined ones (e.g., white sugar, white flour, white rice and instant oats) and the products made from them (e.g., breakfast cereals, white breads, biscuits, pies, cakes, desserts, sweets, ice-cream, soft drinks), can result in a rapid rise in blood sugar because far more sugar is released into the bloodstream than is needed for energy. This in turn causes the pancreas to release insulin, whose job it is to remove sugar from the bloodstream.

If during this process the blood-sugar level falls too quickly or becomes too low, the adrenal glands are stimulated and adrenaline is released. With an increase in adrenaline comes an increase in breathing rate.

Symptoms of these phenomena may include feeling dizzy, shaky, agitated, anxious, confused, fatigued, depressed, short of breath and congested with mucous. Hunger and cravings for more blood sugar–spiking carbohydrates can follow, and a rollercoaster ride of fluctuating blood-sugar levels accompanied by an assortment of symptoms can ensue.

Some people have a strong reaction to a high-starch/high-sugar meal; others may just feel below par with a vague sense of unease or fatigue. Although the release of adrenaline is your body's natural response to maintain equilibrium, your adrenal glands have to enact this emergency procedure every time you eat a lot of sugar and/or sugar-forming foods. This is very stressful to your adrenals, your breathing and your body as a whole.

Swings in blood sugar, and therefore in breathing, are moderated when sufficient protein foods with naturally occurring fat are eaten in the same meal as carbohydrates.

Protein and fat are digested more slowly and they slow down the release of sugar into the blood, avoiding the quick changes in blood-sugar levels that lead to over-breathing. They also contribute valuable nutrients, increase satiety, which makes us feel full sooner and for longer, and provide more enduring energy.

In the modern diet, however, protein foods with their naturally occurring healthy fats are often low in comparison to starch-rich, sugar-rich carbohydrates. Protein with naturally occurring fat is found in meat, fish, chicken, cheese and eggs and is also found in nuts, seeds and avocados.

HOW WOULD YOU RATE YOUR DIET?

Grab a pen now and write in Table 22.1 (page 180) everything you had to eat in the last two days. Include drinks, sugar in tea and coffee, each food that made up your meal, and what was on your toast and sandwich.

Using a highlighter, mark all the things that are sugary (added sugar, soft drink, sweets, cake, jam, fruit juice – but not fruit) or high in starch (potato, corn, breakfast cereal, cake, bread, pasta, rice).

Then have a look at the relative proportions of these foods versus the protein, fat and low-starch carbohydrates (fruits and most vegetables) in each meal or snack. Is your diet skewed towards blood sugar–spiking foods?

TABLE 22.1: MEAL COMPONENTS

	Yesterday	Today
Breakfast		
Morning tea		
Lunch		
Afternoon tea		
Dinner		

Take notice of how you feel after a typical meal. After lunch does your nose block up? Do you feel tired or sleepy, or 'foggy', anxious, agitated, or bloated yet hungry again an hour or so later? Or are you energetic, calm, focused, satisfied and refreshed? Notice how you sleep after different evening meals. Did you snore? How many times did you wake?

Our bodies are simply not designed to process large amounts of sugar and refined grains. Consuming them can have a detrimental effect on your breathing and your nervous system. Instead of a fit, calm, lean machine, you may end up a tired, fraught, overweight snorer – on a machine. Many years of observing this among people with breathing disorders shows a pattern. Noisier breathing, snoring and disrupted sleep are more likely to follow an evening meal where hefty amounts of pasta, rice, bread and potatoes crowd out fresh vegetables, protein and natural fats. Low energy and difficulty staying alert at work are more likely to be a problem after a high-starch/high-sugar lunch. You may find yourself nodding off at your desk, falling asleep in a meeting or even snoring on the job.

If you wish to avoid the afternoon energy slump, try swapping a potato, white bread, rice or pasta–based lunch for a lunch of some protein (e.g., chicken, tuna, eggs, legumes), avocado and non-starchy or salad vegetables; or perhaps a meat and vegetable soup or casserole. You may be pleasantly surprised by how much more staying power you have. When you do have bread, watch the proportion in relation to protein foods and vegetables and choose whole-grain sourdough breads.

> *Bronnie made some changes. She substituted her cereal-and-toast breakfast for a tomato and mushroom omelette and snacked on a small handful of nuts and fruit instead of the usual bag of potato crisps and a bagel. Dinner was meat and three veggies, just like Grandma always cooked. The change was instant – her nose was clear, she didn't have that horrible agitated feeling after a meal, she didn't fall asleep after lunch and Bronnie had the best night's sleep she'd had in decades.*

Including some protein, like nuts and hard-boiled eggs, at each meal and in your snacks can help stabilise your blood sugar, your breathing and even your mood, and prevent triggering the blood sugar–over-breathing reaction.

> *Jim came to a breathing course at the urging of his wife. Judy was exhausted from poor sleep due to Jim's thunderous snoring. Jim too was suffering, disturbed by several overnight toilet visits, and waking with a dry mouth, sore throat, blocked nose and feeling completely unrefreshed. He was nodding off at his desk at least four afternoons a week.*
>
> *Jim arrived for his third session with a big smile on his face – Judy had said that last night was her first full night's sleep in decades. Judy had even wondered if Jim was still alive as he had been so quiet during the night. However, the next day Judy said he was snoring again – although it was intermittent and the decibel rating was lower. When I asked what he had had for dinner, the answer was, 'Pasta and garlic bread last night'. The 'good' night before, it was steak and vegetables.*

INDIVIDUAL DIFFERENCES

People vary in their reaction to different foods and food combinations. You may already be aware of foods that you must not eat due to gluten intolerance, allergic or hypersensitivity reactions, enzyme deficiencies or other discomfort, but also try to identify those that worsen your breathing. Keeping a food diary may help. Discuss your response to different foods with your doctor. This is especially important if you are diabetic or pre-diabetic. A nutritional therapist may sometimes be needed to help you implement appropriate changes in your diet.

HEALTHY PEOPLE – TRADITIONAL EATING

Today, our hospitals and doctors' waiting rooms are full of people with poor nutritional status. Rarely is it diagnosed. They are also full of people who have dysfunctional breathing – also rarely diagnosed. So what should we eat? Who and what should we believe?

It is certainly confusing with all the conflicting advice regarding diet, and I don't proclaim to be an expert. However, as with breathing, the concept of staying with what has stood the test of time and is natural for the human body resonates with me. We are designed to breathe 4–6 litres of air per minute; we are designed to eat a selection of clean, fresh, whole, natural plant and animal foods. We would do well to acquaint ourselves with, and eat according to, the common principles of the nature-based diets of 'traditional' populations who had little chronic disease and often lived to over 100 years of age.

Our food culture has changed most dramatically over the last 60 years. With powerful advertising campaigns, addictively tasty, highly processed artificial foods have become normalised. These foods are convenient, fast and cheap. Being sick, though, is not cheap. Whatever money you might save now by eating cheap processed foods you may well end up paying many times over in healthcare costs. Most of us are happy to spend a little extra to buy quality clothes, a nice car or a multi-function mobile phone. If it does cost more to eat well, isn't it better to pay a little more to the grocer and less to the doctor?

Back to the future

Your great-grandparents were much less likely than you are to be obese, snore or have sleep apnoea; or, for that matter, suffer from asthma, diabetes, irritable bowel disease, celiac disease or cancer. If they were like mine (born in the mid-1800s), they ate fruit and vegetables in season, and a variety of whole grains. They drank the milk and ate the meat of pasture-raised animals that lived a peaceful existence; they ate the eggs and meat of chickens that wandered about the backyard indulging in their natural pickings. They ate real butter on fermented sourdough bread. My great-grandparents lived well, and lived into their 80s. While we wait for definitive answers regarding the many nutritional controversies that plague our times, we can learn from our ancestors. You could ask yourself these questions: 'Is what I am about to eat actually whole, natural food?' 'What has happened to it between farm and table?' 'Is my body likely to be able to digest this food, and is there real nutrition in it?' And my favourite, 'Would my great-grandmother recognise it as food?'

Remember, if it's processed, in a package, with a long use-by date and has unpronounceable ingredients, then it is probably not one to choose.

We may not be able to change our genetics or some aspects of our life circumstances, but we can choose to eat well, we can choose to breathe well, and we can teach our children well.

MAKING CHANGES

Having worked out which foods you consume or which eating habits you have that may be affecting your breathing and your health, try changing just one habit or reducing one or two foods each week, otherwise the transition to healthy eating can be overwhelming.

It is beyond the scope of this book to adequately cover nutrition in all its aspects. Advice from a nutritionist is recommended for those with diabetes and other blood-sugar disorders, and those whose diet or digestive processes have been inadequate for quite some time.

ACTION STEPS FOR HEALTHY EATING
- Eat only when you are hungry; stop when satisfied.
- Maintain an appropriate weight.
- Sit down and slow down when eating.
- Allow two to three hours between eating and going to bed.

Food choices to help look after your breathing:

1. Eat fresh, whole, natural plant foods, grown in healthy soil.
2. Choose whole-foods from healthy animals raised with care, on nutrient-rich green pasture.
3. As much as possible, purchase organic and locally grown foods.
4. Eat adequate (but not excessive) protein at each meal.
5. Avoid sugar and excessive amounts of grains.
6. Learn how to properly prepare grain foods to improve digestibility.
7. Include naturally fermented foods in your diet.
8. Avoid additives, preservatives and fake foods.
9. Avoid processed, refined and denatured foods.
10. Avoid refined and hydrogenated vegetable oils including margarines, and the foods containing them.
11. Limit caffeine consumption; avoid alcohol or caffeine within three hours of bedtime.
12. Favour foods your great-grandmother would recognise.

CHAPTER 23

Water and breathing

Being sufficiently hydrated is important – after all, about 60 per cent of our body weight is attributable to water within our cells, tissues, organs, blood and other body fluids. The water in our body is involved in the relay of chemicals and nutrients around the body and in and out of our cells. It helps regulate our body temperature, helps us eliminate toxins, and keeps our skin and mucous membranes moist.

We maintain hydration by ingesting fluids, and by using water contained in our food, and water that is produced in our cells during metabolism. We dehydrate through sweating, breathing, urination and excretion. Dehydration is an issue for many snorers and sleep apnoea sufferers, who often complain of waking up thirsty and with a dry mouth and throat. Having to lever your tongue from the roof of your mouth with a spoon in the morning is not a great way to start the day!

HOW MUCH WATER SHOULD WE DRINK?

The amount of water you need depends on several factors, including your diet, your state of health and level of physical activity, and the climate. All foods contain water. Some foods are 'water-rich', such as lettuce, cucumber and watermelon. You need more fluids on a hot day and when involved in strenuous or sustained exercise in hot, dry conditions. In general, the more you sweat, the more you need to drink. Thirst is an indicator of the body's need for water but not always a reliable one, particularly in the elderly in hot weather.

It is customary to hear nutritional experts and health and fitness practitioners recommending that we drink eight 250 ml glasses of water a day to stay properly hydrated. However, rigorous scientific proof to support (or contradict) this advice is lacking, and the origin of this ubiquitous dictum is shrouded in mystery.

While urban legends abound, a few critical things about water in the body are often overlooked. Unbeknown to many, the amount of fat in your diet and the way you breathe also play a part in hydration. A big part!

Critical to cell hydration is the fat content of food – water in our cells is actually derived from the metabolism of fats. Fats, especially saturated fats, render much more water during metabolism than do carbohydrates or proteins. When our diet is fat-deficient, we can become dehydrated.[24.1]

BAD BREATHERS LOSE LOTS OF WATER

Water levels in the body are also affected by the way you breathe. Water, as water vapour, exits with the gases from your lungs when you breathe out. There is more water vapour in the exhaled air (6.2 per cent is water vapour) than there is in the air that you breathe in. (The percentage of water vapour in the air varies from a trace in desert regions to about 4 per cent over oceans.) This means water is being lost from the body through breathing. Thus how you breathe is an important consideration in the hydration debate as water loss is high in over-breathers.

The normal volume of air to breathe per minute is around 5 litres. People who breathe heavily, snore heavily or have asthma could be breathing 15 litres a minute. Some people breathe even more. The more air you breathe, the more water vapour you lose on your breath. Breathing 5 litres per minute, you will lose approximately 320 ml of water over a day. Breathe at 15 litres per minute and over the course of a day you lose around 1000 ml (1 litre) of water. This is a significant difference. Bad breathers are high water losers. Several parents have commented to me how much more condensation there is in the morning on the window next to their asthmatic child's bed than next to that of a sibling without asthma.

If you mouth-breathe, then your water losses are even greater, as your nose has special design features to help retain some of the water vapour that is breathed out from your lungs. When people reduce over-breathing, they soon experience less mouth dryness, less thirst, and less sticky mucous. The *need* for water will then be less, with thirst generally being a more reliable indicator.

Breathing rate is also important when considering water needs and losses during exercise. A marathon runner whose resting breathing rate is 9 litres per minute and who mouth-breathes when running loses a lot more water on his breath than a 5 litre/minute baseline breather who runs with his mouth closed. The runner who mouth-breathes is also likely to lose more water through heavier sweating. (Excessive sweating is a common symptom of hyperventilation and a body under stress.)

> Rhett, a first-grade rugby player, used to sweat continuously for two hours after a game, necessitating several showers. He was thirsty and drank a total of 2 litres of water during the game, at half-time and in the first hour after the game.
>
> After breathing training, he found he was able to nose-breathe for a fair part of the game and his after-game sweating time reduced to ten minutes. The only water he took during the game was to rinse his mouthguard and he needed only 400 ml after the game to satisfy his thirst. (In fact, that was beer not water!) For Rhett, breathing efficiently meant much less moisture loss on the breath and less stress on his body. This was evidenced not only by the greatly diminished sweating, but also the absence of asthma symptoms. He went from needing sixteen puffs of his asthma reliever during a game to zero. By breathing less, he lost less water vapour and less carbon dioxide – a natural bronchodilator – on his breath.

How someone breathes is a very important element to consider in the debate over how much water we should be drinking. The eight glasses a day directive (and more if exercising) is only going to suit some people – it may not be enough for some, and could be excessive to the point of harm for others.

TOO MUCH OF A GOOD THING – THE OVER-HYDRATION RISK

Drinking too much water can prove to be dangerous by diluting and depleting important minerals. The minerals and electrolytes in your body fluids help transmit electrical impulses for the proper functioning of your heart, nerves and muscles. Serious electrolyte imbalance can, in its most extreme form, lead to cardiac arrest.

The hazards of over-hydration were highlighted by the publication of research into why hikers were becoming seriously ill, or in some cases dying, on the gruelling Kokoda Trail in Papua New Guinea.[24.2] (Four Australians died on the Kokoda Trail in 2009.) The evidence suggested that in the Kokoda situation, with its high availability of drinking fluids, *exercise-associated hyponatraemia* as a consequence of over-hydration was the problem, rather than dehydration. Hyponatraemia – low levels of sodium – is sometimes referred to as 'water intoxication'. The research indicated the best approach was to drink water according to thirst, rather than loading up ahead of thirst. It also found no evidence that sports drinks could prevent exercise-associated hyponatraemia.

It is also important to be aware that drinking water just before or with meals dilutes your stomach acid, which may lead to digestive difficulties.

IN SUMMARY

The 'eight glasses a day or dehydration' mantra is a modern phenomenon. So many people won't go anywhere these days without taking their water bottle with them and sipping frequently. This is not to discount that some people may need it, and benefit by it, but it should not be seen as a 'rule'.

A large portion of the population over-breathe, and eat a highly processed and poorly balanced diet. All these factors contribute to dehydration. Addressing over-breathing and diet is a far healthier approach to remaining hydrated than just drinking more water in an attempt to compensate.

ACTION STEPS TO HYDRATE YOUR BODY

- Breathe through your nose, including during exercise.
- Breathe correctly – at the optimal rate and volume.
- Eat a balanced, fresh whole-food diet.
- Drink water according to need or thirst (and more in hot weather).

CHAPTER 24

A typical five-day program experience – and beyond

The following is an example of what a heavy snorer with mild sleep apnoea may experience while learning and practising the nine healthy breathing habits over a five day period, and beyond. It is based on the many experiences I have observed in my clinical practice over the last twenty years.

DAY ONE

Attention is given to breathing and posture throughout the day, with spot-checks every hour. This reveals a greater tendency to gulp air through the mouth than was first thought. Previously unnoticed sighing and upper-chest movement are also discovered. By maintaining focus on breathing, by the end of the day the instances of mouth-breathing are less, and posture is better. Situations that were triggering mouth-breathing (concentration, walking, showering) and slumped posture (working at the computer, watching television, chatting at the dinner table) are identified. After slowing the pace of walking in the day to help with nose-breathing, by evening nose-breathing feels more like second nature already. Extra pillows are used in bed.

DAY TWO

There are fewer disturbances and toilet visits during the night and less mouth dryness is noticed on waking. Four ten-minute practice sessions of nose-breathing and diaphragm-breathing while sitting in the coathanger posture are done – one before getting dressed, one on the bus, one while waiting for a meeting to start, and one just before bed. Frequent check-ups on breathing and posture are performed throughout the day.

The percentage of time nose-breathing has increased. Occasions of mouth-breathing are noted (showering, for example). The short breath hold exercise is used to suppress or compensate coughing, yawning and sighing. Walking with nose-breathing is much easier but stairs and hills still need to be taken slowly.

DAY THREE

Waking up is earlier than usual and there is a greater feeling of refresh-ment. Partner reports breathing is generally quieter during sleep, there is less restlessness, and no leg twitching and kicking in bed were noticed. Less use of the short breath hold exercise – coughing, yawning and sigh-ing are less frequent today.

Four ten to fifteen minute practice sessions of nose–diaphragm breathing are done as well as using nose–diaphragm breathing during walking. There is noticeable improvement in walking upstairs. Breath-ing feels lighter and easier. Others have commented that it is quieter. No mouth-breathing detected. After reading the chapter on the food–breathing connection some adjustments to diet are made. Bedtime is earlier due to feeling a little tired.

DAY FOUR

Slept well, no disturbance; no toilet visit; woke early and refreshed. Part-ner reports breathing is slower and quieter – even silent at times. Snoring that was heard was softer, through the nose, and brief.

Nose-breathing is the order of the day and likely of the night as well, as mouth and throat are no longer dry on waking. Diaphragm-breath-ing feels much more natural. Consistently good results for posture and breathing check-ups.

The hibernation diaphragm-breathing exercise is introduced into each of the four practice sessions; now concentrating more on diaphragm-breathing during activities and walking. Use of short breath holds to suppress erratic breathing is rarely needed. Increased awareness of breathing during speech; slowing down and practising inhaling through the nose. Energy much improved and sustained all day.

DAY FIVE

Partner reports no snoring heard. Review of Breathing Pattern Self-assessments and symptoms on Symptom Tracker shows significant improvement. Continue four practice sessions a day: one on waking, one just before bed, and the other two blended into the day's events. Care taken to start out slowly and be mindful of relaxed nose–diaphragm breathing during brisk walking and short periods of jogging and cycling at the gym. Greater ease and enjoyment of exercise is experienced. Continued awareness of breathing control during speech and increased awareness of others' poor breathing patterns!

Based on my clinical experience, average improvement over a five-day period tends to be around a 60 per cent reduction in the total Symptom Score for breathing-related symptoms. This includes significant improvement in nasal congestion and energy levels, less awakenings and gasp/ snort episodes, and an expectation that a bed partner would be reporting less disturbed sleep along with quieter and more even breathing. Many of my clients have been given no-snoring status by their bed partner by the fifth day.

We can't say for sure what is happening with sleep apnoea – a repeat sleep study is needed for that – but apnoea is far less likely to occur in the absence of snoring and heavy breathing. (See Chapter 25 – Working with your doctor.)

For some snorers the reported change may have been less but is often still a welcome downgrade to 'non-divorceable' snoring. For those who are using CPAP, signs of improvement such as less breathlessness, nasal congestion and dizziness and better exercise capacity are usually seen in the daytime. I have found that for some people who have had severe sleep apnoea for many years it can take a few weeks until they start to feel 'normal' again. It is extremely rare for there to be no change reported.

BEYOND DAY FIVE: CONSOLIDATION AND MAINTENANCE

It is also rare for anyone to have completely normalised their breathing within five days. Yes, they may have taken the sharp edge off a breathing pattern problem, but further improvements and consolidation of the changes are important. This can be achieved by continuing with daily practice sessions, and by being mindful of your breathing throughout the day, including during activity.

The practice sessions can be blended into your day. You can 'hibernate' on the bus, in the train, and even while you watch television, especially the mind-numbing variety. It can be helpful to think of yourself as a work in progress. Hopefully by now you look forward to the ten, fifteen or twenty-minute practice before bed because of the quality sleep that has become your reward.

I recommend that you continue some formal practice as long as your breathing pattern, energy levels and breathing-related symptoms continue to improve. By being physically active and applying good breathing practices in every aspect of your daily life, you should be able to gradually reduce the amount of formal practice you do and not only maintain the improvements you have, but improve further over time. Eventually, healthy breathing can become completely automatic. You do need, however, to continue to monitor your breathing. It's a health insurance check-up. I recommend you make use of the additional Assessment columns in Tables 4.1, 4.2 and 4.3 (pages 19, 26, 30–31).

To have your tidal and minute volumes measured, you will likely need a referral to a hospital respiratory laboratory. They might also check your alveolar 'end tidal' carbon dioxide level. A breathing educator may be able to estimate the degree to which your breathing has normalised by checking your alveolar carbon dioxide level with a capnometer or via a special breath-hold test.

Even for those with irreversible factors contributing to their snoring and apnoea – such as emphysema/COPD or anatomical abnormalities like physically blocked noses, overly large tongues, small jaws or narrow faces – breathing training can still be of benefit through improving the mechanics, efficiency, rhythm and control of breathing.

Those with more severe conditions, those whose snoring and sleep apnoea is complicated by other illnesses, those whose improvements fall short of the ideal, and those who wish to take their breathing improvement to the next level are recommended to work with an experienced breathing retraining teacher. (See Chapter 27 – Taking it further.)

If symptoms return

The exercises need to be reinstated if you notice a return of signs and symptoms – for example, during a stressful period or illness. This is where referring back to your Breathing Pattern Self-assessments and Symptom Tracker can prove valuable. This situation may be preventable in the future if you identify and address any triggers or lifestyle factors responsible for deterioration in your breathing, such as poor diet and continue to improve your baseline breathing pattern and recondition your breathing set point.

A return of symptoms may also occur if for example you have a very stressful day, have a large, heavy meal with two glasses of wine just before bed and then sleep flat on your back with your mouth open. Breathing volume will go up and carbon dioxide levels drop. Such a 'relapse' should only be temporary if you identify the culprits that affected your breathing and do what you need to get good breathing back on track.

CHAPTER 25

Working with your doctor

MEDICATIONS, DEVICES, APPLIANCES AND BREATHING RETRAINING

Many people are dependent on medications, devices and appliances to address the symptoms and conditions associated with their sleep-disordered breathing. At the same time, many find they are obliged to live with the inconvenience and/or side-effects these treatments may in turn cause. It is a rejection, intolerance or failure of these treatments that brings many people to the breathing retraining approach. There are others, however, who are comfortable and well managed on their treatment but seek a more natural approach for travel or social reasons, or wish to address daytime breathing-related issues like stuffy nose, irritable cough, shortness of breath, panic attacks and reduced exercise capacity.

Breathing retraining offers a wonderful opportunity to take back control of your breathing and improve the quality of your life. It is empowering, but with that power comes responsibility. When you change something as fundamental as the way you breathe, regular monitoring by yourself and your doctor is essential.

Participants in breathing retraining programs are requested not to alter or cease medication usage or CPAP or oral splint usage without first consulting their doctor, no matter how well they feel their condition is controlled. If you are working with a breathing teacher, they will look at various indicators to make recommendations for the timing of a review. If you are working on your own at improving your breathing habits, your Breathing Pattern Self-assessments and Symptom Trackers can be valuable tools in guiding you as to when it is time to see your doctor for review.

Your doctor can reassess your condition, monitor the effects of the changes in your breathing pattern and determine your requirements for prescribed treatments for your snoring, sleep apnoea and associated conditions if and when necessary. This will often require a repeat sleep study to ascertain the degree of any improvement or change in your condition. Your dental professional also needs to be consulted if you have been prescribed an oral appliance.

A fully integrated approach is the best for you. It is ideal if there is communication and collaboration between all medical and allied health professionals and educators involved in your care.

It is possible that prescribed treatments may no longer be required. This has been the experience of many people who have learnt to breathe correctly. However, withdrawal of prescribed treatments needs to be a medically monitored and supervised process.

CHANGING NEEDS – REAPPRAISAL OF PRESCRIBED APPLIANCE USE

Though CPAP and oral splints are generally prescribed for life, it is recognised that making significant habit and lifestyle changes such as losing weight, giving up smoking, doing more exercise and even a reduction in stress levels can reduce the severity of snoring and apnoea and significantly reduce the need for these appliances.

When people retrain their breathing, enabling them to consistently breathe through their nose and to breathe more regularly and quietly at the correct rate and volume, this also represents a marked change of habit that is likely in the majority of cases to influence the status of a person's snoring and sleep apnoea. When you have evidence of significant change and improvement it could be time to visit your doctor to request a review of your situation. Two examples are given below.

Example one: Someone not (currently) using CPAP or oral splint

If following diagnosis of sleep apnoea, and while you are considering or being assessed for CPAP or an oral splint, you undergo a breathing retraining program, here are what some signs of improved breathing could be:

- You feel better and have more energy; you remain alert and have no drowsiness during the day; your breathing is easier during exercise; nasal congestion is reduced or gone; you sleep with your mouth closed; you have stopped waking yourself with a snort or gasp.
- Your partner reports that you no longer disturb them at night; they have observed no apnoea episodes; they notice significantly less or no snoring; they notice your breathing is slower and more regular.

Example two: Someone using CPAP

If you already use CPAP, you cannot assess your natural breathing while you are sleeping with the machine on. However you (or others) may still see some indicators of significant change that warrants seeing your doctor. These could be:

- Improvement in daytime symptoms such as blocked nose, breathlessness and fatigue.
- Observation by your partner or companion that you no longer snore when you fall asleep without your CPAP on (for example, on the couch, or in bed before you put your mask on, or when you throw it off during the night, or when you are travelling).
- You have undisturbed sleep, wake refreshed, have improved concentration and energy, and have no symptoms of excessive tiredness or drowsiness in the day following a CPAP-free night (for example while travelling).
- You start to find the flow or pressure of air from your CPAP mask too strong or 'confronting' as you work at improving your breathing. This may indicate that the pressure you require now is less than before breathing retraining. Pressure settings must be appropriate to ensure effectiveness and comfort.
- If you have one of the latest CPAP models that provide data on the number of times the machine is activated through apnoeas, and you have evidence that the number of apnoeas is reducing.

> *Mike had been on CPAP comfortably for many years, on a setting of 8.5 cm H2O. He came to see me as he wished to travel overseas and was concerned that there could be situations where it would be difficult to use his machine. After three days of breathing training he became very uncomfortable on the machine – he said it felt like he was 'fighting against it'. He spoke to his CPAP consultant and the machine's pressure was reduced, and he then slept comfortably on CPAP again – for another three nights. After then battling the machine for two hours one night he took the mask off, rolled over onto his side and slept the rest of the night without the machine. He breathed through his nose, woke without any nasal congestion or dry mouth and had energy throughout the next day. His wife who was a light sleeper did not notice any snoring or apnoea. Mike was then advised to see his doctor and have a repeat sleep study to confirm the status of his apnoea condition.*

If you have been following the program outlined so far and haven't already done so, take the time now to complete another daytime and sleep breathing pattern assessment (Chapter 4, Tables 4.1 and 4.2, pages 19 and 26). How does your breathing now compare to before – nose- vs mouth-breathing, diaphragm vs upper-chest breathing, regular vs erratic breathing? Has the frequency of yawning and sighing changed? Have the number of waking, gasping or choking episodes changed? What is your respiration rate and resting heart rate now compared to before?

With improvements to your breathing, as you move closer to physiologically normal breathing, you are less likely to experience snoring and sleep apnoea. People with physiologically normal breathing by definition cannot have snoring and sleep apnoea. They could, though, have a (usually) temporary problem with snoring if their breathing got disturbed again one night by, for example, a late and heavy meal consumed with a few wines and followed with sleeping on their back.

You might also like to complete another assessment column on your Symptom Tracker (Table 4.3, pages 30–31). Has there been a change in the amount of mucous, number of headaches, energy and concentration levels, overnight toilet visits, restless legs, anxiety and need for a daytime nap, and so on?

Some clients of mine set up audio and video recording of their sleep to get feedback. There are even mobile phone applications that can measure snoring. While these options provide useful information, for a quantitative objective assessment, you need an overnight sleep study.

If your doctor has had little exposure to breathing retraining (as apart from general breathing exercises), it may help a lot if you show them your Breathing Pattern Self-assessments and Symptom Tracker when you go for review. In effect, they provide a progress report. This will help them see what the program involves and what your response has been. Your doctor is particularly likely to be pleased to see improvement in your condition if you have previously rejected surgical or appliance-based approaches or if they have not worked for you.

If it appears your sleep apnoea condition has changed significantly, your doctor may suggest or agree to a follow-up sleep study to give an objective evaluation.

Reducing CPAP use

When patients on CPAP have undertaken breathing training in the hope that they may be able to do without CPAP, issues such as a trial period without CPAP or at a reduced pressure need to be discussed with the doctor and be medically supervised. For those whose breathing has improved through breathing retraining or other means like weight loss, a doctor may consider gradually reducing the pressure and/or the time on CPAP while monitoring the patient's signs and symptoms and doing a repeat sleep study at some stage. Some of the later models of CPAP automatically adjust the pressures delivered according to the patient's (changing) requirements and have computer chips that can give valuable information such as the number of apnoeas experienced.

Ideally, a reduction in CPAP pressure or use, or a trial period without CPAP, should be done at a time when the person is relatively stress and commitment free, such as a holiday period, and during a time when they do not need to drive. This is so they can observe their response without putting themselves or others at risk while they do activities that need focus and concentration.

In some states of Australia, driving licences are sometimes endorsed to require use of CPAP. A change to such an endorsement on a licence would require a satisfactory result on retesting in a sleep laboratory.

If at any time during a reduction in CPAP use a person experiences increased or excessive daytime sleepiness while sitting, reading, watching television, or during conversation, then it is vital they return to the use of CPAP at a level where they were symptom-free, and of course speak to their doctor. They need to be certain there is no tendency to lose concentration or inappropriately drift off to sleep during the day. If warranted, the process could be tried again after further sustained efforts to improve breathing.

In the case study in the Appendix B, you can read about one severe sleep apnoea sufferer's before, during and after experiences, including repeat sleep studies.

LONG-TERM RESPONSIBILITY

Those who, in consultation with their doctor, have reduced CPAP pressure or stopped using a treatment need to keep in mind that breathing retraining is a self-management approach for breathing – *not a snoring or sleep apnoea cure*. Should your breathing pattern deteriorate, your symptoms may return or new symptoms may arise. So continue to close your mouth, sleep on your side, watch your food choices and alcohol consumption and most importantly, mind your breathing.

Stress has a huge impact on breathing. Therefore when people are under stress – situations can include job loss, intense physical exertion, grief or other strong emotion, illness, surgery or infection – your breathing may become deeper and/or faster again, putting you at risk of a return of symptoms.

To avoid this, you should keep an eye on your breathing pattern every day, watch out for symptoms, and check your heart rate on waking. Then you can take action accordingly to maintain yourself in a symptom-free range.

If your dysfunctional breathing is not corrected, or is not correctable for any reason, you will need to return to the use of CPAP or an oral splint. Whatever management or treatment option you have taken, should your symptoms get worse or return, see your doctor.

CHANGING NEEDS – REAPPRAISAL OF PRESCRIBED MEDICATION

Just as sleep apnoea requires monitoring so that treatment is adapted to a person's changing needs, so too do associated conditions such as high blood pressure (hypertension), heart conditions, diabetes, depression and other disorders for which medications are prescribed. When your breathing improves several things may happen:

- Your body may become more efficient at metabolising or excreting a medication.
- Your body may become more sensitive to a medication.
- The body function that the medication is supplementing or replacing may normalise.
- The symptoms that the medication was treating may lessen or be eliminated.

This means that if you substantially change your breathing, there is a possibility that your requirements for medications can change, and research has borne this out.[25.1–25.4] Therefore, reassessment of your medication needs by your doctor is very important.

It has been long known that making lifestyle changes can affect a person's requirements for medications and treatments. For example, if you are overweight, losing weight and exercising more may lower your blood pressure and blood-sugar levels and increase the sensitivity of your cells to insulin.

In summary, breathing retraining can be a wonderful tool to help you take back control of your breathing, improve your sleep, your health, and the quality of your life. However, when you change your breathing, it is vital that you see your doctor for review and advice regarding any serious health conditions you have and any changes in prescribed treatments and medication.

CHAPTER 26

Hold-ups to improvement

If your progress towards better breathing and better sleep is slow, use this list to help identify issues that may be promoting or reinforcing disordered breathing, or preventing you from making progress. I have found the most common issues to be:

1. Laziness – neglecting to observe breathing and practise the exercises.
2. Persistent, unconscious over-breathing and mouth-breathing.
3. Fully exhaling – emptying or pushing air out of your lungs.
4. Slumped posture.
5. Holding your stomach in all the time.
6. Insufficient physical exercise.
7. Mouth-breathing and poor breathing control while exercising.
8. Sleeping flat on your back with your mouth open.
9. Over-heating in bed.
10. Over-sleeping.
11. Large meals near bedtime.
12. Overeating.
13. Eating foods that increase your breathing rate.
14. Excess alcoholic, caffeinated and sugary drinks.
15. Smoking and second-hand smoke.
16. Exposure to a lot of stress.
17. Gasping inhales through your mouth during speech.
18. Not persevering long enough with breathing retraining.
19. An anatomical, structural, mechanical or muscle function problem that needs treatment.

20. Presence of chronic inflammation or infection in your body, such as in the nose, sinuses, tonsils, mouth or teeth, or as tinea or candida.
21. A medical condition you have, and/or medication(s) you take which affect your breathing/increase your breathing rate.
22. Being so sleepy that your ability to concentrate and retain information is poor.

What to do? If you have identified an area where you think change is still needed and it is something you can address yourself, give it a try. You could revisit the action steps for those healthy breathing habits that are not yet second nature or get help from a breathing teacher. If symptoms of sleep apnoea are still interfering with your daily life, consult your doctor.

In the case of points 19–22, you need to see the appropriate health professional(s) for investigation and treatment. For point 19, those who work synergistically in this area include orofacial and ENT surgeons, sleep physicians, dentists, orthodontists, breathing retraining teachers, physiotherapists, speech pathologists, orofacial myologists and osteopaths. In the case of point 22, you must see your doctor urgently as you likely need CPAP or other medical treatment in order to get enough quality sleep to allow you to learn and make whatever changes in your breathing and lifestyle that you can.

If your sleepiness is only after meals or at the end of a day's work I also suggest you read and practise the suggestions in this book at a time of day when you are most alert. Most of my training sessions for people with sleep-disordered breathing were held at 7.30 a.m. – this worked better than after lunch or after work. Even the most skilled breathing teacher can't teach someone who is asleep!

When there is a lot more than bad breathing habits going on, progress with breathing training may be slow or limited. This may be the case with certain heart conditions or when breathing is mechanically compromised through severe obesity, severe COPD, hyperinflation of the lungs, musculoskeletal deformity of the chest wall, weakness or paralysis in breathing muscles, or anatomical abnormalities in the throat and windpipe. CPAP, or another form of assisted ventilation, for life may be essential. However, if breathing training can improve efficiency and control to any degree in the day, it can make breathing more comfortable and improve exercise capacity.

FINDING TIME TO PRACTISE

If finding time to practise is the problem, please review the suggested practice times and ways to blend better breathing into your normal day. If you can find the time to read a novel for 30 minutes or polish your car, you can find the time to practise better breathing.

A small amount of effort and application will be handsomely rewarded. You service your car so it will last the distance. Give care of your breathing priority too. After all, breathing is something you need to keep doing for the rest of your life. Doing *it* well will serve *you* well.

CHAPTER 27

Taking it further

The basics of breathing retraining as they appear in this book can be safely self-taught and can deliver wonderful results within a very short period of time. So often I have seen simple instruction in breathing awareness, posture and nose-breathing produce dramatic improvements in total Symptom Scores. Many students reported either fewer or no signs of snoring and gasping episodes just by establishing nose-breathing and side-sleeping as a habit.

While this book provides valuable information and practical instruction, it is still ideal to undertake breathing retraining with a skilled teacher. A book provides general information; a teacher can tailor that information to the specific needs of an individual and take into account the broader circumstances, such as complicated health conditions. It is certainly beyond the scope of this book to try to match what a good teacher can do.

THE BENEFITS OF WORKING WITH A BREATHING RETRAINING TEACHER

Undergoing breathing retraining with a teacher may assist you to go faster and further in normalising your breathing. When a teacher observes your breathing and posture, and takes your personal health history into account, they can choose the best approach for you from among the various exercises and techniques available. Their supervision ensures exercises are done correctly and, where appropriate, they can use intensive training and 'stronger' techniques. They can estimate the degree to which your breathing has normalised by checking your alveolar carbon dioxide level with a capnometer or via a special breath hold test.

Even when working with a teacher, not all students are able to completely normalise their breathing. There may be anatomical or pathological reasons for falling short of the ideal, or they may stop their practice at the point of partial normalisation. However, any improvement can make a tremendous difference to quality of life.

A study has shown that three months after beginning practice of the Buteyko method of breathing retraining, the average minute volume for a group of chronic asthmatics had reduced significantly from 14 litres per minute to 9.6 litres per minute.[27.1]

Although this indicates that a degree of over-breathing was still occurring, nonetheless, the results recorded were extraordinary: an average 71 per cent reduction in symptoms, 96 per cent reduction in use of bronchodilators and 49 per cent reduction in steroid preventative medication.

At the three-month point, the Buteyko group were a long way from where they started, and a long way ahead of the control group, who were on a conventional asthma management regime and who did not improve in any aspect and were unable to reduce their medications.

FINDING A BREATHING RETRAINING TEACHER

As defined in Chapter 10, breathing retraining is the specific discipline where the goal is to normalise each aspect of the breathing pattern.

Although the popularity of breathing retraining is spreading, as a specific field of healthcare it is still relatively unknown. Within the public health system you may find breathing retraining programs, but they are far from being universally available. In most westernised countries breathing retraining is available privately from individual teachers and practitioners. With time, as the scope, effectiveness and benefits

> **THIS BOOK IS NOT A BUTEYKO METHOD COURSE**
>
> This book is not a self-help version of the Buteyko method of breathing retraining. You cannot apply the principles and exercises in this book and say that you have 'done' or 'learnt' the Buteyko method. It does have its foundation principles and primary aim (to normalise breathing) in common with the Buteyko method but does not contain the full array of practices that defines the Buteyko method.

of breathing retraining becomes more widely known and documented, I believe it will become more broadly available to the public as an integral part of mainstream medical and hospital practice and community health initiatives.

In fact, small changes are already occurring. For example, in the United Kingdom, New Zealand and the Netherlands some hospitals and general medical practices now offer Buteyko-based breathing retraining.

An internet search will help you locate professional bodies and affiliated and non-affiliated breathing retraining teachers to learn something about their philosophies, their approach, and the rigour of their training.

CHAPTER 28

Conclusion

Breathing retraining works, and together with simple lifestyle changes can prevent much of the day-to-day suffering endured by so many poor breathers. And it is never too late to change. One of the first breathing training clients I had was nearly 80. She volunteered herself for a television news story because she wanted to let other people know that 'you *can* teach an old dog new tricks'.

I have several hopes for this book and the first is for you. I hope that *Relief from Snoring and Sleep Apnoea* inspires in you a lifelong commitment to breathing correctly, and that with that change you go on to enjoy a lifetime of peaceful, refreshing sleep, abundant health and vitality, and a wonderful quality of life.

In addition, knowing first-hand what it is like to watch children struggle to breathe, I hope that the message of this book spreads far and wide to parents everywhere so that they can know the value and importance of correct breathing for their children's health, development and wellbeing.

I wish you silent, restful nights, and a long and healthy life. I wish for you the very best, *for every breath you take.*

APPENDIX A

Researching breathing retraining for sleep apnoea

At the time of writing, breathing retraining has not been clinically trialled specifically for sleep-disordered breathing. However, there is a large body of anecdotal evidence supporting its effectiveness, and people with snoring and sleep apnoea now form the largest category that breathing retraining teachers see.

Results from a retrospective survey on breathing retraining for sleep apnoea are very promising. Buteyko Institute practitioners who participated in the 2010 survey on behalf of the Buteyko Institute of Breathing and Health (BIBH) had collectively taught over 11 000 clients with sleep apnoea. A majority of practitioners (73 per cent) estimated that over 95 per cent of clients had improved sleep after completing a course in breathing retraining.

In addition, symptoms such as snoring, headaches and restless legs also improved in the majority of clients according to the practitioners' estimations.* The BIBH has sent the survey report to sleep researchers and discussions are underway about conducting clinical trials.

---

* *Sleep Apnoea and Breathing Retraining: To what extent is the Buteyko Institute Method of breathing retraining effective for sleep apnoea? A survey of Buteyko Institute practitioners' experiences with clients suffering from sleep apnoea. Birch M. 2012. The report is available at www.buteyko.info/ latest_buteyko_news.asp?newsid=27*

APPENDIX B

Case study – a new lease of life

The case study below illustrates what can happen when you follow a planned and supervised breathing retraining process. I chose this particular case because it was recent and because this person had received the documentation from her three sleep studies.

I wish to make it clear that Juliana (not her real name) did a full course of breathing retraining with an experienced Buteyko-trained practitioner – someone other than myself.

Please be advised that this case study can only represent the outcome of the breathing retraining process (Buteyko Institute Method) for this particular person. With sleep-disordered breathing there are many factors peculiar to an individual that will affect the outcome. The outcome achieved in Juliana's case cannot necessarily be achieved for others.

JULIANA, 55-YEAR-OLD HEALTH PROFESSIONAL

Juliana was diagnosed with severe obstructive sleep apnoea at age 54. The diagnosis was made almost by chance when she consulted a specialist dentist for another matter. This dentist also specialised in diagnosis of sleep apnoea and made oral devices to treat sleep apnoea. He prescribed an 'at home' sleep study for her after reviewing her sleep apnoea information questionnaire, and because of her excessive daytime sleepiness and her husband's concerns that she sometimes stopped breathing at night and then seemed to struggle to start breathing again.

When the results came back, the dentist deemed her condition too severe to be treated with an oral device, so she commenced CPAP and was also advised to consult with an ENT (ear, nose and throat) surgeon.

The sleep study showed that Juliana stopped breathing on average 68 times an hour during her dreaming sleep stage, (REM sleep), and 21 times an hour on average overall. Her longest apnoea was almost one minute. Although her condition improved over a couple of months on CPAP, Juliana did not like the idea of sleeping with a CPAP machine for the rest of her life. While waiting for the appointment with the surgeon, she heard about a Buteyko breathing retraining program and decided to join the next course.

During the week of the breathing course, Juliana continued to use the CPAP machine. On the second day of the course she attended a routine two-hour choir practice and experimented with inhaling only through her nose while singing. Juliana was delighted and amazed to find that after two hours of singing, she felt as fresh as when she started – she had none of the usual giddiness or hoarseness, nor any difficulty breathing. Juliana felt that now she could be on the right track to learning what the underlying breathing problem was and how to improve it.

Her appointment with the ENT surgeon was scheduled for three days after the breathing course finished. He found Juliana had no need for surgery. Juliana discussed the breathing course and her wish to have a trial period off CPAP with this surgeon (and later with the dentist who initially identified her sleep apnoea). Both the surgeon and the dentist were agreeable to monitoring her condition with follow-up sleep studies. Juliana was willing to go back onto CPAP if her sleep apnoea and daytime sleepiness persisted in spite of breathing retraining. She was also willing to consider an oral device depending on the outcome of her breathing retraining.

Juliana stopped using CPAP on the day of the consultation with the surgeon. Throughout the trial period she diligently practised the breathing exercises and continued to pay attention to training herself to breathe only through her nose in all situations, day and night.

After two weeks, during which time Juliana did not use CPAP, she had a repeat sleep study (at home). This second study showed significant improvement – the number of 'events' had reduced to an average of just five per hour and her oxygen levels were much better. Snoring was significantly less. The diagnosis was revised from severe to mild obstructive sleep apnoea. Conservative management was recommended and CPAP no longer considered necessary. From her breathing practitioner's point of view Juliana was considered 'a work in progress' and further work on improving her breathing was required.

Four months later, she had her third sleep study. This was conducted at a sleep clinic. This time, Juliana got a clean bill of health – no evidence of central, obstructive or mixed apnoeas, even though she spent more than half the night sleeping on her back.

Juliana says she now feels like she has a new lease of life – she is no longer sleepy during the day, does not need CPAP and, although she was never medically diagnosed with a daytime breathing problem, she has found to her surprise that it is just so much easier to breathe now all the time, whether she is working, exercising, singing or just sitting around.

Frequently asked questions

Q: *How could breathing retraining in the day work when snoring and apnoea are night-time problems?*

A: The way you breathe during sleep is a reflection of the way you breathe when awake. People who snore and have sleep apnoea invariably breathe incorrectly during the day as well as night. They have faulty breathing habits, and those habits can be changed. While breathing is automatic, you can also consciously vary it – you can practise breathing at the correct rate, rhythm and volume during the day, which resets the the 'drive to breathe' centre in your brain, to deliver quieter, softer, more regular breathing at night. Sometimes on the first night!

Q: *Is breathing retraining any use when my nose is nearly always blocked?*

A: Yes. Noses are often 'blocked' as a result of irritation, dehydration, and inflammation – all side-effects of chronic over-breathing, the faulty breathing habit most often seen in snorers. When you learn to breathe correctly, airway irritation reduces. In twenty years of breathing retraining, I have rarely seen a nose that won't, at least partially, clear within the first five minutes of changing a poor breathing pattern – not even smashed-up footballers' noses, of which I have tackled a few.

Q: *I get panicky when I shut my mouth – is breathing retraining even possible for me?*

A: Many people cannot tolerate 'forcing' nose-breathing by simply trying to keep their mouth closed, or through wearing a chin strap, as they become claustrophobic or feel as though they are suffocating. Breathing retraining gradually 'reconditions' you, so you can achieve comfortable nose-breathing at your own pace.

———

Q: *I have been told I have a deviated septum/floppy soft palate/large tongue/small jaw and I need surgery. How could breathing exercises help?*

A: Consider this: unless you have had facial injuries, you likely have had the same anatomy – the same shaped nose and upper palate and the same sized jaw and tongue – all your adult life. If you are 45 now and chronically snore, but did not at age 28, it is more likely the *way you breathe* has changed over the years than your tongue has grown larger or your septum more deviated. Likely you breathe faster or heavier now than you used to. If so, there is a very good chance that breathing retraining exercises will help. That's not to say that having a bent or narrow nose and a receded jaw does not put you at greater risk of snoring and apnoea. It's just that the way you breathe is a critical element in determining how much trouble they will cause you (see Chapter 6).

———

Q: *How can breathing retraining help me when the problem is my throat collapsing?*

A: Your throat doesn't just collapse through bad luck, bad genes or because you are overweight. There is always a component of dysfunctional breathing present and it's highly likely that it is contributing. Those great big breaths that get sucked in fast during a bout of heavy snoring can create a suction force sufficient to bring the walls of the throat closer together. Breathing retraining can help restore a stable, even breathing pattern and reset a 'breathing over-drive'.

Q: *Can breathing retraining help me? I can't tolerate CPAP and I am desperate to get a good night's sleep.*

A: Breathing retraining offers welcome relief to those who cannot tolerate sleeping with a face mask and a continuous positive airway pressure (CPAP) machine. While CPAP is generally very effective, research indicates that over 50 per cent of people suffering from sleep apnoea are non-compliant with the recommended therapy. Thankfully breathing can be retrained – you can learn to breathe correctly again.

Q: *If breathing retraining is so good, why did my doctor only recommend surgery/dental splints/CPAP machines to me?*

A: There is a general lack of knowledge and interest in breathing pattern dysfunction. Most doctors are not well informed about the principles of breathing retraining, and observation and assessment of a patient's habitual breathing pattern is not part of standard medical diagnosis. The extent of 'dysfunctional' breathing in the population is grossly underestimated. Most doctors have simply not considered breathing retraining as an option for their patients.

Breathing retraining is a logical, scientific and conservative approach to the management of breathing disorders. Your doctor should be no more reluctant to suggest you improve your breathing habits than to recommend other self-help approaches such as stopping smoking, avoiding alcohol, losing weight, getting fit and sleeping on your side with your mouth closed. Not only is addressing disordered breathing patterns common sense, it also makes economic sense.

Q: *How long does it take to feel a difference with breathing retraining?*

A: People usually notice less nasal congestion and quieter and easier breathing within hours (or even just minutes). Better sleep is often reported right from the first night. 'The best sleep in decades' is a frequent comment.

Q: *I learnt breathing exercises before and felt dizzy/breathless/tired after them. Why would breathing retraining exercises be any different?*

A: If the breathing exercises you learnt involved big, deep in-breaths with full exhales, particularly if by mouth, then likely you caused a shortfall in carbon dioxide in your blood. This can result in some blood vessels narrowing and reducing the amount of oxygen that gets through to your brain and muscle cells. Thus dizziness, breathlessness and fatigue may occur.

The difference with a breathing retraining program as described in this book is that you are taught to breathe normally – at the correct rate and volume – so that you keep your blood gases in balance. This is essential in allowing the oxygen in your blood to actually get to the cells where it is needed. This is vastly different from a focus on getting as much oxygen into your lungs as possible.

Q: Does it take a lot of time? I don't have time to do breathing exercises.

A: Why not? You are breathing all the time aren't you? You can make changes in your breathing any time in the day – while you watch television, walk to the car, sit on a plane or a train. This is one of the advantages for busy people of breathing retraining over other exercise programs.

Q: Do I have to stop other treatments?

A: No, you can practise breathing correctly while you continue to use medications, machines, appliances, and so on. In fact, improving your breathing can make it easier to tolerate an oral splint or a face mask and CPAP machine. Ultimately though, if you can return your breathing to how it was when you did not snore – that is, get your breathing softer, slower, quieter and more regular again – your requirement for these corrective treatments may change and then you can discuss your situation with your doctor.

Glossary

CPAP	continuous positive airway pressure
COPD	chronic obstructive pulmonary disorder
CSA	central sleep apnoea
ENT	ear, nose and throat (specialist)
OSA	obstructive sleep apnoea
REM	rapid eye movement
TMJ	temporomandibular joint
UARS	upper airway resistance syndrome

adenoids – gland-like tissue at the back of the nasal passage.

alveoli – the little air sacs in the lungs where gas exchange occurs.

anaerobic metabolism – the creation of energy through the combustion of carbohydrates when there is insufficient oxygen for energy production.

anatomy – the science of studying the structure and shape of an organism.

apnoea – cessation of breathing.

arousals – an abrupt change from deep sleep to a lighter stage of sleep, which may or may not lead to waking up.

Bernoulli effect – states that the faster the flow (of air), the greater the partial vacuum or negative pressure created on the walls of the passage.

Bohr effect – states that the release of oxygen from the haemoglobin in the blood into the tissues is dependent on the level of carbon dioxide in the blood .

breathing-control centre – see 'respiratory centre'.

breathing pattern disorder – a combination of different signs and symptoms that may be seen when there is disturbance in normal breathing function.

breathing retraining – the specific discipline where the primary goal is to normalise each aspect of the breathing pattern for all situations.

capnometer – a device used to measure the amount of carbon dioxide in the exhaled breath.

central sleep apnoea – when breathing repeatedly stops during sleep because the brain temporarily stops sending signals to the muscles that control breathing.

chronic obstructive pulmonary disease (COPD) – a lung disease; it includes chronic bronchitis (a long-term cough with mucous) and emphysema (involves damage to the alveoli). The main symptom is breathlessness.

deviated septum – a crooked partition in the nose.

diaphragm – the major breathing muscle.

dysfunctional breathing – abnormality in breathing; impairment in the breathing function.

hard palate – the hard part of the roof of the mouth; see 'palate'.

hypercapnia – carbon dioxide level above normal.

hyperventilation – breathing an amount of air that is excessive in relation to metabolism and which creates a deficiency of carbon dioxide.

hypocapnia – carbon dioxide level below normal.

hypopnoea – under-breathing; breathing that is shallower or slower than normal.

hypoventilation – insufficient ventilation to meet the body's oxygen requirements and to eliminate the appropriate amount of carbon dioxide.

hypoxia – deficiency of oxygen.

insomnia – inability to sleep or difficulty in falling or staying asleep.

lactic acid – a chemical that is formed when sugars are broken down for energy in the absence of sufficient oxygen.

metabolic rate – the rate at which energy is used by the organism.

metabolism – the chemical processes occurring within a living cell or organism that are necessary for the maintenance of life.

minute volume – the total volume of air breathed per minute.

mixed sleep apnoea – a combination of obstructive and central apnoea.

obstructive sleep apnoea – a condition where breathing repeatedly stops or significantly decreases during sleep because of a narrowing or obstruction in the upper airway, typically in the pharynx.

occlusion (in dentistry) – the alignment of the teeth of the upper and lower jaws when brought together.

over-breathing – breathing an amount of air that is excessive in relation to metabolism and which creates a deficiency of carbon dioxide.

palate – the palate, in the roof of the mouth, consists of the hard palate and the soft palate. The hard palate at the front of the mouth contains bone; the soft palate at the back does not contain bone. The soft palate is movable, consisting of muscle fibres sheathed in mucous membrane. From the soft palate hangs the uvula.

paradigm – a view accepted by an individual or a society as a clear example, model, or pattern of how things work.

pH – a measure of the acidity or alkalinity of a solution.

pharynx – the wall of the throat behind the nose and tongue.

physiology – the science that deals with the mechanical, physical and biochemical functions and processes of the body.

polyps – small sac-like growths of inflamed mucous membrane in the nose or sinuses.

polysomnograph – recording of a number of physiological functions and events during sleep.

respiratory centre – the 'breathing-control centre', the special group of cells in your brainstem that regulates the rate and depth of breathing to keep the carbon dioxide concentration in your arterial blood at the optimal level (set point) so that all bodily processes function well. It determines the signals to be sent to the respiratory muscles.

respiration rate – the number of complete breaths taken per minute.

restless legs – a feeling of uneasiness and restlessness in the legs, generally of an evening and after going to bed, but can occur during the day .

rhinitis – inflammation of the mucous membranes of the nose.

signs – any indication of a condition that can be objectively observed.

sinusitis – inflammation of the sinuses.

sleep-disordered breathing – An abnormal pattern or quantity of breathing occurring during sleep.

smooth muscle – sometimes called involuntary muscle. A type of muscle found in many places in the body, including the walls of the airways and blood vessels.

soft palate – the soft part of the roof of the mouth; see 'palate'.

solar plexus – the area of the upper abdomen above the navel and below the lower end of the breastbone.

symptoms – subjective experiences; something consciously affecting the patient.

tidal volume – the volume of air inhaled and exhaled at each breath. Normal tidal volume is 500 ml.

tonsils – glands, situated in the throat.

uvula – the punching bag–shaped piece of tissue hanging from the back of the soft palate.

Venturi effect – describes how a flow of air accelerates as it enters a narrowed passage.

Chapter reference and resource materials

CHAPTER 1

1.1 'Global surveillance, prevention and control of chronic respiratory diseases: a comprehensive approach'. Jean Bousquet and Nikolai Khaltaev editors. World Health Organization 2007. http://www.who.int/gard/publications/GARD%20Book%202007.pdf. Accessed 14 April 2012.

1.2 'Effectiveness of nasal continuous positive airway pressure (nCPAP) in obstructive sleep apnoea in adults'. National Health and Medical Research Council, endorsed 2000. www.nhmrc.gov.au/_files_nhmrc/file/publications/synopses/hpr21_0.pdf. Accessed 3 October 2011.

1.3 'Sleep Apnea and Sleep'. National Sleep Foundation (USA). www.sleepfoundation.org/article/sleep-related-problems/obstructive-sleep-apnea-and-sleep. Accessed 28 September 2011.

CHAPTER 2

2.1 'Sleepy Driver Danger' Walker, F. *Sun Herald*, 11 February 1996. Retrieved from http://www.driverslicenses.com.au/drivers-licenses-articles/1996/2/11/sleepy-driver-danger/ Accessed 19 March 2012.

2.2 'Assessing Fitness to Drive'. Austroads. March 2012. p 105. http://www.austroads.com.au/images/stories/AFTD_reduced_for_web.pdf. Accessed 19 March 2012.

2.3 The Effect of Snoring and Obstructive Sleep Apnea on the Sleep Quality of Bed Partners. Beninati W, Harris CD, Herold DL, Shepard JW. Mayo Clinic Proceedings October 1999; 74(10): 955-958.

2.4   'US couples seek separate bedrooms', BBC News, 12 March 2007. http://news.bbc.co.uk/2/hi/americas/6441131.stm accessed 19 March 2012-03-19

CHAPTER 3

3.1   'Respiration during sleep in normal man'. Douglas NJ, White DP, Pickett CK, Weil JV and Zwillich CW. *Thorax* November 1982; 37(11): 840–844.

3.2   'Respiratory physiology: breathing in normal subjects'. Krieger J. In *Principles and Practice of Sleep Medicine*. Kryger MH, Roth T, Dement WC, eds. 2005; Elsevier Saunders: Philadelphia.

CHAPTER 5

5.1   'Control of breathing in obstructive sleep apnoea and in patients with the overlap syndrome'. Radwan L, Maszczyk Z, Koziorowski A, Koziej M, Cieslicki J, Sliwinski P, Zielinski J. *Eur Respir J.* 1995; 8(4): 542–545.

Resources for Physiological Norms

Review of Medical Physiology. Ganong WF. 6th ed. 1973; Lange Medical Publications.

Human Physiology. Vander A, Sherman J, and Luciano D. 5th ed. 1990; McGraw Hill, New York.

Principles of Anatomy and Physiology. Tortora GJ and Grabowski SR. 8th ed. 1996; Harper Collins College Publishers. P. 728.

Physiology of Disease Processes. Anderson Price S and McCarty Wilson L. 4th ed.1992; Mosby Year Book Inc.

CHAPTER 6

6.1   'Hypocapnia'. Laffey JG and Kavanagh BP.*N Engl J Med*. 2002; 347: 43–53.

6.2   'Treatment of mast cells with carbon dioxide suppresses degranulation via a novel mechanism involving repression of increased intracellular calcium levels'. Strider JW, Masterson CG and Durham

PL. *Allergy* 2011; 66: 341–350.

6.3   'Control of breathing in obstructive sleep apnoea and in patients with the overlap syndrome'. Radwan L, Maszczyk Z, Koziorowski A, Koziej M, Cieslicki J, Sliwinski P, Zielinski J. *Eur Respir J.* 1995; 8(4): 542–545.

6.4   'Con: Sleep apnea is not an anatomic disorder'. Strohl KP. *Am J Respir Crit Care Med.* 2003; 168: 271–272.

6.5   'Is chronic hyperventilation syndrome a risk factor for sleep apnea?' Coffee JC. *Journal of Bodywork and Movement Therapies.* 2006; Part 1, 10: 134–146.

6.6   'Is chronic hyperventilation syndrome a risk factor for sleep apnea?' Coffee JC. *Journal of Bodywork and Movement Therapies* 2006; Part 2, 10: 166–174.

6.7   'Effects of nasal positive-pressure hyperventilation on the glottis in normal sleeping subjects'. Jounieaux V, Aubert G, Dury M, Delguste P and Rodenstein D. *Journal of applied physiology* 1995; 79 (1).

6.8   'Hyperventilation–apnea syndrome: a new clinical entity?' Moldovanou I and Tcheban A. *Biological Psychology* August 1995; 41(1): 93–93.

6.9   'A possible mechanism for mixed apnea in obstructive sleep apnea'. Iber C, Davies S, Chapman RC and Mahowald MM. *Chest* 1986; 89: 800–805.

6.10   'Effects of mouth opening on upper airway collapsibility in normal sleeping subjects'. Meurice JC, Marc I, Carrier G and Series F. *Am. J. Respir. Crit. Care Med.* 1996; 153 (1) 01: 255–259.

6.11   'Hypocapnia and increased ventilatory responsiveness in patients with idiopathic central sleep apnea'. Xie A, Rutherford R, Rankin F, Wong B and Bradley TD. *Am J Respir Crit Care Med.* 1995; 152: 1950–1955.

6.12   'Crossing the apneic threshold: Causes and consequences'. Dempsey, Jerome A. 2004.Julius H. Comroe Memorial Lecture – Experimental Biology, Washington DC. April 2004. Physiology in Press; published online on 30 November 2004 as 10.1113/expphysiol.2004.028985.

6.13   'The ventilatory responsiveness to carbon dioxide below eupnoea as a determinant of ventilatory stability in sleep'. Dempsey JA, Smith CA, Przybylowski T, Chenuel B, Xie A, Nakayama H and Skatrud JB. *J Physiol.* 2004; 560: 1–11.

6.14   'Effects of inhaled carbon dioxide and added dead space on idiopathic central sleep apnea'. Xie A, Rankin F, Rutherford R and Bradley TD. *J Appl Physiol.* 1997; 82: 918–926.

6.15   'Low-concentration carbon dioxide is an effective adjunct to positive airway pressure in the treatment of refractory mixed central and obstructive sleep-disordered breathing'. Thomas RJ, Daly RW and Weiss JW. *Sleep* 2005; 28: 12–13.

6.16   'Alteration in obstructive apnea pattern induced by changes in oxygen and carbon-dioxide-inspired concentrations'. Hudgel DW, Hendricks C and Dadley A. *Am Rev Respir Dis.* July, 1988; 138(1): 16–9.

6.17   'Mechanisms of obstructive sleep apnea'. Hudgel, DW. *Chest* 1992; 101(2): 541–9.

6.18   'Effect of continuous positive airway pressure on central sleep apnea and nocturnal PCO2 in heart failure'. Naughton MT, Benard DC, Rutherford R and Bradley TD. *Am J Respir Crit Care Med.* 1994; 150: 1598–1604.

CHAPTER 7

7.1   'Hyperventilation syndrome: A diagnosis begging for recognition' (Topics in Primary Care Medicine). Magarian GJ, Middaugh DA and Linz DH. *West J Med.* 1983; 138: 733–736.

7.2   'Hyperventilation: the tip and the iceberg'. Lum LC. *Journal of Psychosomatic Research* 1975; 19: 375–383.

7.3   *Breathe Well, Be Well.* Fried R. 1999; John Wiley & Sons.

CHAPTER 9

9.1   'Effect of continuous positive airway pressure on central sleep apnea and nocturnal PCO2 in heart failure'. Naughton MT, Benard DC, Rutherford R and Bradley TD. *Am J Respir Crit Care Med.* 1994; 150: 1598–1604.

9.2   Research in sleep and ventilation. Researcher: Research and Development New, March 2003 edition. Royal Brompton and Harefield NHS Trust.

9.3   'Effectiveness of nasal continuous positive airway pressure (nCPAP) in obstructive sleep apnoea in adults'. National Health and Medical Research Council, endorsed 2000. www.nhmrc. gov.au/_files_nhmrc/publications/attachments/hpr21_0.pdf. Accessed 3 October 2011.Pp. 27–28.

9.4   'Adherence to continuous airway pressure treatment for obstructive sleep apnea: implications for future interventions'. Weaver TE and Sawyer AN. *Indian J Med Res.* 2010; 131: 245–258.

CHAPTER 10

10.1.   'A controlled study of a breathing therapy for treatment of hyperventilation syndrome'. Grossman P, De Swart JC and Defares PB. *J Psychosom Res.* 1985; 29: 49–58.

10.2   'Buteyko breathing techniques in asthma: a controlled trial'. Bowler SD, Green A, Mitchell CA. *MJA* 1988; 169: 575–578.

10.3   'The effect of physiotherapy-based breathing retraining on asthma control'. Grammatopoulou EP, Skordilis EK, Stavoli N, Myriantheps P, Karteroliotis K, Baltopoulos G and Koutsouki D. *Journal of Asthma* 2011; 48: 593–601.

10.4   'Didgeridoo playing as alternative treatment for obstructive sleep apnoea syndrome: randomised controlled trial'. Puhan MA, Suarez A, Lo Cascio C, Zahn A, Heitz M and Braendli O. *BMJ* February 2006; 332 (7536): 266–70.

10.5   Borg B, Doran C, Giorlando F, Hartley MF, Jack S, Johns DP, Wolfe R, Cohen M, Abramson MJ. The Buteyko method increases end-tidal CO_2 and decreases ventilatory responsiveness in asthma, in The Australian and New Zealand Society of Respiratory Science Inc. Annual Scientific Meeting. (2004). http://anzsrs.org.au/asm2004abstracts.pdf

10.6   Austin et al. Buteyko Breathing Technique Reduces Hyperventilation-Induced Hypocapnia and Dyspnoea. Am. J. Respir. Crit. Care

Med. 2009; 179: A3409

CHAPTER 19

19.1 *The Melba Method*. Dame Nellie Melba. 1926; Chappell & Co. p 10.

CHAPTER 23

23.1 'Dry Skin'. Cowan T. The Weston A Price Foundation: Ask the Doctor 30 June 2000. Retrieved from www.westonaprice.org/ask-the-doctor/dry-skin.

23.2 'Over-hydration "hazard for Kokoda hikers"'. Rose D. *Sydney Morning Herald* 6 March 2011. Retrieved from http://news.smh.com.au/breaking-news-national/overhydration-hazard-for-koko-da-hikers-20110306-1bj97.html.

CHAPTER 25

25.1 'Breathing control lowers blood pressure'. Grossman E, Grossman A, Schein MH, Zimlichman R and Gavish B. *Journal of Human Hypertension* 2001; 15: 263–269.

25.2 'Slow breathing improves arterial baroreflex sensitivity and decreases blood pressure in essential hypertension'. Joseph CN, Porta C, Casucci G, Casiraghi N, Maffeis M, Rossi M and Bernardi L. *Hypertension* 2005; 46: 714–718. doi: 10.1161/01.hyp.0000179581.68566.7d

25.3 'Buteyko breathing techniques in asthma: a controlled trial'. Bowler SD, Green A, Mitchell CA. *MJA* 1988; 169: 575–578.

25.4 'Buteyko breathing technique for asthma: An effective intervention'. McHugh P, Aitcheson F, Duncan B and Houghton F. *N Z Med J*. 2003; 116 (1187): U710.

CHAPTER 27

27.1 'Buteyko breathing techniques in asthma: a controlled trial'. Bowler SD, Green A, Mitchell CA. *MJA* 1988; 169: 575–578.

Learning resources

All information here is supplied in good faith, but you should also make your own enquiries and seek professional guidance if necessary before purchasing any of the products or services or undertaking any process, therapy or treatment.

AUDIO AIDS TO LEARNING
BREATHING EXERCISE INSTRUCTION AUDIO
If you prefer to learn through listening, you may benefit from our special package that includes an audio recording of breathing exercise instructions – to listen to during your practice times.

Go to Store at: www.BreatheAbility.com.

WORKBOOK
Download the free workbook containing the Breathing Pattern Self-assessment Tables, the Symptom Tracker, and the Observation Checklist.

Go to Store at: www.BreatheAbility.com.

WEBSITES
AUTHOR WEBSITE
www.BreatheAbility.com

OTHER USEFUL WEBSITES
www.austat.org.au
Australian Society of Teachers of the Alexander Technique

www.buteyko.info
Buteyko Institute of Breathing and Health

www.westonaprice.org
The Weston A. Price Foundation

RECOMMENDED READING

Nutrition and Physical Degeneration. Dr Weston A. Price. 6th ed. 2004; Price–Pottenger Nutrition Foundation. ISBN 0-87983-816-7

Nourishing Traditions. Sally Fallon with Mary Enig. 1999; New Trends Publishing, Inc. ISBN 0-9670897-3-5
This book has an excellent overview of nutrition, teaches food preparation and has dozens of recipes. It is both a cookbook and an educational aid.

Changing Habits, Changing Lives. Cyndi O'Meara. 2007; Penguin Group Australia. ISBN: 978 0 14 300652

Shut Your Mouth and Save your Life (1870). Catlin, G. 2009 reprint; Kessinger Publishing. ISBN 1104304562, 9781104304560

Acknowledgements

Firstly, I want to thank my husband, children, extended family and friends for their support and encouragement over the years I have been researching and writing this book. My special thanks to Karen St Clair for her patient reading of drafts, for lending her editing skills to them, and most of all for her wisdom and clear vision that has helped keep me on-purpose throughout the process.

My appreciation also to my book and chapter reviewers: Helen Best, Mary Birch, Kay Coombe, Greg Brackenreg, Maria Dight, Peter Donnelly, Anne Farrell, Jennifer Harris, Victoria Kleeberg, Dr Patrick McHugh, Sharon Moore, Paul O'Connell, Christine Ritchie, Torben Ronholt, Dr Michael Ryan, Michael Stenning, Peter Thompson and Glenn White. The book is manifestly better because of your thoughtful input and constructive suggestions in your various areas of expertise. I want to especially thank Dr Ross Walker whose achievements as a clinician, author and educator remain a great source of admiration and inspiration.

Thank you to all the team at Penguin, including Alex Ross for the cover design, Laura Thomas for the text design and Bridget Maidment, my editor, for the skill and polish she applied to the manuscript. A special thank you to Julie Gibbs who first saw the promise of my work, and to my publisher, Andrea McNamara for her skill and guidance.

I would also like to thank Anthony Calvert whose illustrations captured the essence of the book, and my agent Fitzroy Boulting for his advice and support. Finally, I am grateful to all my clients whose enthusiasm, commitment and willingness to take responsibility for their health inspired me to produce this work.

**NEED A DYNAMIC SPEAKER AT YOUR NEXT CONFERENCE OR BUSINESS EVENT –
ONE WHO CAN LEAD PEOPLE TO ACHIEVE INSTANT RESULTS?**

Do you want your participants to leave your event inspired and feeling better? That's what Tess wants too and she has an uncanny ability to make it happen.

Tess Graham is a sought after Keynote Speaker with a powerful message. She is a world authority on what it takes to get a quiet, restful night's sleep, to wake refreshed and have energy and focus all day long. For nearly two decades, Tess has delivered informative, relevant and practical programs that have enabled thousands of people to breathe better, sleep better, and be better, in so many ways . . . starting immediately.

This is because when Tess speaks about breathing, people change. They change what they think about breathing, and they change the way they breathe. When they change the way they breathe their experience of sleep changes. So too does their capacity for work, life and play.

To book Tess for your next conference or business event, go to
www.BreatheAbility.com

Informative – Relevant – Practical